DR. DONSBACH'S

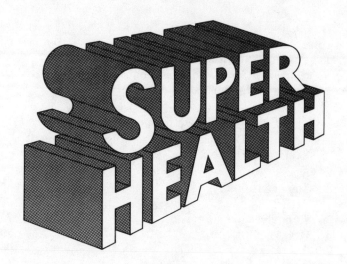

SUPER HEALTH

BY

KURT W. DONSBACH, Ph.D.

Donna Burgard

Health is Wealth

TABLE OF CONTENTS

INTRODUCTION

Having been involved in various writing efforts over the past many years, I'm very much aware of the importance of a title descriptive enough to enthuse a potential reader into picking up the book. I take no credit for originality in my work since I consider myself a gatherer of facts already researched but, in some instances, not adequately presented or written in a style easily understood and applied to daily life.

The concept of *SUPERHEALTH* is more than just the absence of disease. Too many in our day and age accept minor aches and pains as an interest payment on advancing years. I am not convinced that such signs of deterioration are inevitable or necessary. If we can but accept a concept that I sincerely believe and uphold, we can achieve that feeling of vitality, that extra sparkle in the eye, that extra mental inquisitiveness that can make life a real pleasure to live. That concept simply stated is, "Every disease known to man, not induced by trauma, is related to a disturbance in the chemical balance within one's own body." Upon acceptance of this concept, one merely needs to find his own individual biochemical weaknesses and strengths and use food and nutritional supplementation to enhance perfection of function.

We have too long been fed with almost religious fervor a line of poppycock that would lead us to believe that everyone is a little sick, that a little pain and suffering are normal, that all one needs to do is reach for aspirin, Tums, or if in dire need, rush to the deity that we call doctor and have them miraculously alleviated. The flaw in this approach lies in the fact that the cause of pain is not lack of aspirin, a stomach upset is not due to a lack of a fizz fizz — plop plop alkalizer, and the medicine practiced by our orthodox physicians is primarily elimination of symptoms rather than elimination of causes. By their own admission, over 70% of patients get well regardless of the type of treatment administered if, in fact, any is administered.

This is also a very elemental viewpoint since wellness is defined in medical terminoligy as a lack of disease. Just because you don't feel quite right, or you don't have the energy you feel you should have, is not adequate evidence for the allopathic physician to classify you as being other than normal. Thus, all too many of us go through life without ever experiencing *SUPERHEALTH*.

It is my sincere hope that this book will be of some assistance to those who have the interest and inclination for a better state of life and who wish to try a little different approach. Granted, some of our tenets are controversial, but to the best of my knowledge and experience, they work.

Chapter 1

Positive Nutrition in Action

The study of nutrition involves the relationship of foods and food factors to the health of the human body. In general, the discrepancies in health we are concerned with are due to deficiencies of one or more of the food factors. These food factors can be generally considered to be PROTEIN, FATS, CARBOHYDRATES, FIBER, MINERALS, ENZYMES AND VITAMINS.

The classification of deficiency diseases in medical literature has been discussed largely in relation to the so-called "classical examples," i.e. Beri-Beri (vitamin B-1 deficiency), Pellagra (vitamin B-3 or niacin deficiency), Scurvy (ascorbic acid deficiency) and Kwashiorkor (protein deficiency). These diseases are always produced by extreme dietary environments, being found in their "pure" form only in "starvation" areas of the world or where an individual obviously deviates far from what is considered to be an ordinary diet. They will be seldom, if ever, encountered in the average doctor's practice.

Nevertheless, these rare deficiency diseases are the basis of the teaching in schools and, in most cases, they form the basis of judgment upon which the average doctor reflects his diagnosis and treatment. Actually, these diseases represented only initial discoveries and, as such, provided the stimulus for investigation into a vast variety of deficiency disease possibilities. And, led by visions of new discoveries on this extended horizon, scientists, research workers, and doctors (as individuals) have been actively engaged in uncovering new nutritional entities ever since.

1

Literally, hundreds of thousands of such investigations have been made by these men. This has resulted in a vast accumulation of technical literature — literature which largely gathers dust in scientific libraries. This is understandable because most of the findings were written in a scientific tone and did not lend themselves to practical clinical situations. It is also regrettable because this same literature provides the means of making invaluable contributions towards preventative medicine — a field which almost all will agree is being grossly neglected today in so-called modern medicine.

The purpose of this analytical study will be to dust off the literature, correlate what has been thoroughly researched but often not utilized and present a manual of the nutritional aspects of disease.

NATURE'S LAWS

"You may drive Nature out with a pitchfork, yet she will ever hurry back, to triumph in stealth over your foolish contempt." (Horace) The ancient as well as present day philosophers are well aware of the inexorable force that Nature exerts upon us. We suffer greatly by tampering with her laws and benefit just as greatly by working with these laws. Perhaps in no other field is this more dramatically brought to our attention than in nutrition. Definitive disease results from ignorance, deliberate transgression or circumstantial inability to meet the nutritional needs of the body. Just as definitive a reversal of the disease process is brought about by supplying the body with proper nutrients needed for the process of metabolism.

The beautiful and oft overlooked fact that when one is working with Nature, progress and results can be relatively easily predicted, is a constant source of surprise to one who is consistently using an approach to disease which may be contrary to Nature. Applied Nutrition can offer you an invaluable adjunct to your health practices plus the accompanying benefits of faster results.

CALORIES

Before approaching nutrient groups, it is important to define and understand a term which relates (falsely) nutrition to more minds than any other — CALORIES.

CALORIE: The amount of heat required to raise the temperature of one gram of water one degree centigrade.

In more common measures, we can equate the above with the amount of heat required to raise the temperature of four pounds (two quarts) of water one degree Fahrenheit. It is also readily seen that the term is used only as a measuring index signifying the chemical energy released when a food is metabolized. As a general approximation, the following can be used as physiologic food values:

Protein	4 calories per gram
Fat	9 calories per gram
Carbohydrates	4 calories per gram

It is important to remember that the above table relates to grams of pure food source; in other words you would have to know that amount of each food category in a given food to determine the calories therein represented. It was for this purpose that the caloric charts are included. For easy conversion, remember that each ounce contains approximately 28 grams.

CALORIES DO NOT REIGN IN NUTRITION!

Many charts have been produced regarding the caloric needs of a man or woman. These charts vary from 2,000 to

6,000 calories per day depending upon the type of activity of the individual. Low calorie diets abound — all based on the *theory* that if you take in less calories than your body requires for the type of work you do then you must lose weight. This becomes true only when that caloric intake is drastically beneath requirement levels and, as many thousand dieters will attest, is extremely difficult to maintain. It has been said there are more low calorie diet plans than there are successful followers of such plans.

Perhaps the reason for the rather consistent failure of such diets lies in the body with its extremely complex metabolic processes. Probably the most important fact of body chemistry which relates to this discussion is: "THE ABILITY OF THE TISSUES TO OXIDIZE FAT IS, IN CONTRAST TO CARBOHYDRATES, UNLIMITED." The term "oxidize" means to burn up. Your body burns up *food* to create the energy you need through the process of oxidation. It will only burn up storage fat and protein as a last resort. The fact that the body converts unoxidized carbohydrates to fat which is *stored* thus completes the picture. All low calorie diets are particularly low in fats of any kind but usually recommend copious amounts of vegetables and fruits, both of which are high in carbohydrates.

Fat has a higher satiation factor; you require much less to turn off your appestat than carbohydrates. Thus, even though one gram of fat has more than twice the calories of one gram of carbohydrate, it is readily conceivable that the gram of fat will create a better atmosphere for weight loss than the carbohydrate. This is also the basis of the "Atkins" type diet which has received much attention recently.

CALORIES DO NOT COUNT, BUT THE FOOD FROM WHICH YOU DERIVE THOSE CALORIES COUNT SIGNIFICANTLY.

Protein

Every animal, including man, must have an adequate source of protein in order to grow or maintain itself. Proteins, which yield amino acids, are the fundamental structural element of every cell of the body. Specific proteins and protein derivatives are now recognized as the functional elements in certain specialized cells, glandular secretions, enzymes and hormones. Thus protein well deserves its name, which is of Greek derivation, meaning "OF FIRST IMPORTANCE."

Proteins are among the most complex organic compounds found in Nature and are made up of nitrogen-containing compounds known as amino acids. During the digestion of proteins, hydrochloric acid and other proteolytic enzymes such as pancreatin effectively break down the intact protein molecule into the amino acids which then are absorbed through the intestinal wall. It is important to note that intact proteins are not absorbed — if they should be, serious consequences can occur. Most usual are allergies or allergy-like reactions.

It is appropriate, in light of the above, that every nutritionist concern himself with the status of the digestive functions of a patient when protein intake is being considered. Enzyme supplements are sometimes indicated, and one must be careful not only to use a complete enzyme supplement, but also adequate amounts. A formula containing the following approximate amounts can be given from one to four tablets with each meal:

Betaine Hydrochloride	60mg
Pepsin (l:3,000)	35mg
Pancreatin (4x)	75mg

This formula is for comparative purposes only and, to the best of my knowledge, no such exact formula is available.

However, these three enzymes are the essential ones for protein breakdown. If an enzyme contains these three plus others, it does not in any way detract, but rather enhances the total digestion.

ESSENTIAL AMINO ACIDS

Amino acids are classified as either essential or non-essential. The basic difference is that the non-essential can be synthesized in the body from the essential group, provided that there is an adequate supply of the essential amino acids. A very important fact to remember is: IN ORDER FOR A TISSUE OF THE BODY TO DO A PARTICULAR JOB — CELL GROWTH OR TISSUE SYNTHESIS — ALL OF THE ESSENTIAL AMINO ACIDS MUST BE PRESENT AT THE SAME TIME. A missing amino acid cannot be supplied several hours later and find the other essential ones on the job until all can be assembled.

This is the famous "All or None" law of protein utilization. It emphasizes the need for a variety of protein sources in a meal, particularly if one source is considered an incomplete protein (very low or lacking in one or more of the essential amino acids).

The Essential Amino Acids Are:	Rec. Daily Intake:
Leucine	2200mg
Isoleucine	1400mg
Valine	1600mg
Methionine	2200mg
Threonine	1000mg
Lysine	1600mg
Histidine	800mg
Phenylalanine	2200mg

Tryptophan   910mg
Arginine (can be synthesized by the animal
    organism, but not at a sufficiently rapid rate
    to meet the demands for normal growth
    and repair)

The recommended daily intake listed on the foregoing chart does not reflect what I would consider an adequate amount. Recent research has indicated that protein requirements can fluctuate in a similar fashion to that of Vitamin C — under stress conditions the need may be increased tenfold. However, the chart is valuable in general percentages information regarding the ratio of the essential amino acids in a food or protein supplement.

Another aspect of protein metabolism which can influence the choice of food which might be used as a source is the PROTEIN EFFICIENCY RATIO. Over the years a variety of terms have been used to assign values to protein-yielding foods — Biological Value, Chemical Score, etc. These terms attempt to classify a protein food according to the most limiting essential amino acid contained as compared to a standard — which has been whole chicken egg or casein. The chart below gives some representative foods and their P.E.R.

FOOD	P.E.R.
Egg, chicken	1.0
Milk, human	0.9
Milk, cow	0.7
Muscle, beef	0.7
Soybean meal	0.6
Rice, whole	0.5
Wheat, whole	0.4
Potatoes	0.6
Oats, whole	0.6
Corn, whole	0.4

It will be obvious from the above that certain high quality protein foods (ex. potatoes, whole oats) yield a low quantity of protein per volume consumed, thus should not be depended upon to supply a major portion of the dietary requirement.

PROTEIN REQUIREMENTS

Any quantitative estimate of protein requirement must take into account the quality of the proteins involved. A general rule of thumb has been 1 Gram of protein for every Kilogram (2.2 lbs.) of body weight. This leaves a great deal to be desired since it does not apply to the obese or the emaciated nor does it take into account the extra needs of the growing children, the pregnant woman, or the nursing mother. It can be generalized according to the following chart:

MALE and FEMALE Recommended Daily Protein Intake	
Under one year	3.5 Grams/2.2 lbs.
One to three years	40 Grams
Four to six years	50 Grams
Seven to nine years	60 Grams
Ten to twelve years	70 Grams
Thirteen to twenty years	75 — 100 Grams
MALE — Adult	70 — 100 Grams
FEMALE — Adult	60 — 90 Grams
Pregnant	85 — 100 Grams
Lactating	100 — 120 Grams

Although there has always been controversy regarding the possible benefits or harm of a high protein diet, I personally am of the opinion that the above chart is a rational reflection of the basic needs for protein intake to satisfy the constant demand in the body. We are not only rebuilding muscle and organ cells with this protein, but some of the amino acids play extremely important roles in the formation of hormones, others are used in the creation of enzymes which are then necessary to break the crude protein down into amino acids. HIGH QUALITY PROTEIN IS A REJUVENATOR!

EFFECTS OF PROTEIN DEFICIENT DIET

1. Lowering of hemoglobin levels
2. Increased intra-cellular fluid — Edema
3. Depression of vitamin A levels (lack of transport) protein)
4. Decline in liver enzyme activity
5. Growth retardation
6. Nausea
7. Dizziness
8. Muscular incoordination
9. Retarded spermatogenesis
10. Extreme weakness
11. Cataracts
12. Acid — Alkaline balance deviations
13. Hormone deficiencies — thyroxine, adrenaline, insulin
14. Lowered resistance because of lack of antibodies

There is a widely believed concept that excess protein will overburden the liver and kidneys with metabolic wastes and create such conditions as gout, liver and kidney disease. It is now substantiated that a diet consisting of 100 — 150 grams of protein, 200 or more grams of fat and less than 20 grams of carbohydrates produces an exceptionally healthy body with no high blood pressure, gout, liver or kidney disease. In fact there seems to be no harm from the consumption of 300 grams of protein daily if adequate water

9

is consumed to take care of the urinary wastes. Such a consumption would be very difficult to accomplish but is offered as an example only.

On the other hand, we have rather impressive research indicating that although a high protein intake may not be harmful, it also may not be necessary. A volunteer group of individuals who performed hard physical work daily were put on a comparative low protein diet (40 to 55 grams daily). The published results of this study indicated that a daily intake of 53 grams of protein was sufficient to maintain excellent health without loss of strength. My basic comment on this would be cautionary in nature — Remember that the body needs all the essential amino acids present at one time. Low protein diets often tend to be comprised of incomplete protein foods during some meals, therefore this protein is "lost" as far as metabolic value is concerned. However, there is no question that a good vegetarian who includes adequate amounts of raw seeds and nuts in the diet can lead a very healthy life.

PHENYLKETONURIA

The PKU Syndrome is probably the most well-known of protein abnormalities. It affects children, and if undetected, produces mental retardation and aberrations. These children are unable to convert the essential amino acid, phenylalanine, to tyrosine with resulting high levels of phenylalanine in the serum which is diagnostic of the disease. The condition must be diagnosed within the first month of the baby's life in order to prevent brain damage. The exact mechanism of the brain damage is not known, although it may be due to the lack of tyrosine, considered a non-essential amino acid because of the body's ability to convert the phenylalanine — which in this case it cannot. This disease afflicts 1 out of 10,000 children and can be controlled by the special PKU diet.

10

PROTEIN SUPPLEMENTATION

I must stress that quality is of first importance in your choice of protein supplements. Percentages do not tell the whole story and can be misleading. Multiple source products are preferable due to the better essential amino acid content as a general rule. It must be remembered that concentrated protein contains almost no fibre and thus can be constipating. Recommend additional water intake with them. It may also be wise to use a protein digestant tablet for absorption.

PROTEIN EXCESS

It has been pointed out that the doctor may not only see symptoms of protein deficiencies in his practice, but also those of protein excess in the diet. There is no question that protein can cause toxicity to occur in the body when eaten exclusively to the exclusion of the other important food groups, particularly fats and fibers. Or, if the liver is malfunctioning, the kidneys underactive and detoxifying mechanisms as a whole are weak or overloaded we have a problem. Let me explain.

Proteins are broken down by enzymes in the digestive tract before being absorbed. These digestive acids and enzymes not only break down the protein into amino acids but also help to prevent the multiplication of the bacteria often associated with protein and the putrefactive bacteria associated with undigested proteins. Thus, a breakdown of the digestive secretions allows dangerous bacterial growth in the intestinal tract.

The inclusion of fats in the diet stimulates the production of bile which also acts as a natural laxative. As mentioned before, protein tends to be constipating, again allowing putrefactive bacterial growth. In the same sense, we must include fiber in the diet as a natural antagonist to the putrefactive bacteria because it does not give them time to multiply and be resorbed in the tract. The production of bile is also a natural outlet for the liver to dump unnecessary amino acids out the eliminative route of the feces.

The kidneys also play an important part in protein digestion and utilization. Proteins are acid in nature and the by products of protein metabolism in the body are acid. Most of these are eliminated in the urine as phenols, skatols, uric acid, etc. Thus the importance of proper kidney function is a prime factor in possible protein toxemia.

The liver-kidney cleansing regime outlined later is a must when the signs of protein overload are present — uremia, lassitude, mental torpor.

NUCLEO-PROTEINS

Deoxyribonucleic acid (DNA) and ribonucleic acid (RNA) have been referred to as nucleo-proteins although this is probably not technically correct. These two factors are the responsible entities which determine the rebuilding process of the cell. DNA is the master chemical blueprint for building of new cells and the RNA is the messenger chemical that carries out the DNA's instructions. DNA is literally the cornerstone of the life process. Whenever new cells are required, the DNA sends out RNA molecules to gather the materials to form them.

Life continues normally until the DNA ceases to form RNA after which cell regeneration is seriously inhibited or stopped. When this becomes widespread, death ensues. Although death is the final result, it is now common knowledge that this decrease in production of RNA can lead to decreased function in a particular organ or area which can reflect itself either as acute disease or chronic

12

degenerative disease depending on the organ or gland involved.

A variety of terms have been used to describe the DNA factor — cell determinants, protomorphagens, etc. What really is of interest to the practicing doctor is whether or not it is possible to rejuvenate or stimulate the DNA-RNA functions in the body. It has been rather scientifically determined that the addition of RNA substance to the diet of animals had a certain rejuvenating effect, particularly on memory and thought clarity.

Physicians have for years been injecting liver extracts, expecting and most of the time receiving admirable results in many disorders. Some would like to attribute these effects to the iron and vitamin B Complex factors inherent in liver, but when the same quantities of these substances are used alone, the results are not the same. It has therefore been postulated that animal glandular tissue concentrates in some way transmit specific DNA stimulants which are not explained by their vitamin, mineral or protein content.

Fats

Fats, or lipids, are the most concentrated source of energy in the diet. When oxidized, fats furnish more than twice the number of calories per gram furnished by carbohydrates or proteins. One gram of fat yields approximately nine calories to the body. Perhaps this factor and such erroneous information as the "cholesterol scare" have made the inclusion of fats in the diet a very limited one indeed. Hopefully, this presentation plus the later discussion on cholesterol problems will clear away much of the fog and once again allow this very important nutrient group to attain its rightful place in our diets.

In addition to providing energy, fats act as carriers for the fat-soluble vitamins, A, D, E, and K. By aiding in the absorption of Vitamin D, fats help make calcium available to body tissues, particularly to the bones and teeth. Fats are also important for the conversion of carotene to Vitamin A. Fat deposits surround, protect, and hold in place organs, such as the kidneys, heart and liver. A layer of fat insulates the body from environmental temperature changes and preserves body heat.

Fats prolong the process of digestion by slowing down the stomach's secretions of hydrochloric acid. Thus, FATS CREATE A LONGER LASTING SENSATION OF FULLNESS AFTER A MEAL.

FATTY ACIDS

The substances that give fats their different flavors, textures, and melting points are known as the "fatty acids." There are two types of fatty acids — saturated and unsaturated. Saturated fatty acids are those that are usually hard at room temperature and which come primarily from animal sources (Coconut oil is an exception to this, since it is a vegetable source, but is saturated.) Unsaturated fatty acids, including polyunsaturates, are usually liquid at room temperature and are derived from vegetable, nut, or seed sources, such as safflower, sunflower, corn, and sesame. Vegetable shortenings and margarines have undergone a process called "HYDROGENATION" in which unsaturated oils are converted to a saturated form by chemically forcing the unsaturated oil to accept hydrogen ions. Since the chemical difference between a saturated and an unsaturated fat is the amount of hydrogen ions present, the so-called unsaturated margarines are really quite saturated.

ESSENTIAL FATTY ACIDS

In the past, there have been three fatty acids considered "essential" (since the body could not produce them) LINOLEIC, LINOLENIC and ARACHIDONIC. These have been erroneously referred to as the "Vitamin F" group, but since their action in the body is not that of a vitamin, such terminology is rarely used. Although it was at one time considered that all three of the essential fatty acids could not be produced in the body, it has now become apparent that in the presence of *adequate vitamins and minerals* the body can synthesize linolenic and arachidonic from linoleic. Practically speaking, this should not deter us from using foods which are good sources of these two fats. Let me give you a few reasons why:

1. THE MORE ARACHIDONIC ACID THERE IS IN BLOOD, THE GREATER THE RESISTANCE TO ATHEROSCLEROSIS.
2. CLOT FORMATION SUCH AS SEEN IN CORONARY PATIENTS CAN BE MARKEDLY REDUCED

15

IN A FEW HOURS BY THE ADDITION OF LINO-
LENIC ACID.

3. PROSTAGLANDINS (hormone-like compounds
which help to regulate such diverse reactions as
gastric secretion, pancreatic functions, release of
pituitary hormones, etc.) ARE MADE FROM ARA-
CHIDONIC ACID.

These essential fatty acids are found in all oils to some
degree, but the following will give you the best sources:

Linoleic — Safflower, sunflower, sesame, walnut and
soy oils.

Arachidonic — Peanut oil

Linolenic — Soy oil

Since oils oxidize rather rapidly which then produces
rancidity, it is highly recommended that oils be tightly
capped immediately after use and returned to refrigeration.
Because of this tendency, it is said that margarines,
hydrogenated cooking fats and highly refined commercial
vegetable oils (used in commercial deep fryers) are often
prepared from rancid oils. They can be deodorized, but the
deleterious chemical changes can never be reversed.
BEWARE!

Although butter has been much maligned as food, let us
compare the essential fatty acid content with its common
replacement.

	% of Essential Unsat. Fatty Acids
Butter	4.0 to 6.0
Margarine	2.0 to 5.0

In the very category for which it makes so many claims
(essential unsaturated fatty acids) margarine comes out
second best. Enough said!

RECIPE FOR SUPER BUTTER:

1 lb. butter

2 fl. oz. safflower oil

2 fl. oz. soy oil

2 fl. oz. peanut oil

Allow butter to reach room temperature, put all four ingredients in a blender and mix thoroughly. This mixture will mold into any container when put in refrigerator and has an excellent flavor with super quantities of essential unsaturated fatty acids. I recommend that you buy the small size of these three oils and use them in equal quantities for cooking as well as making your "super butter" recipe. Remember, the smaller the quantity you buy, the less chance you have for it becoming rancid.

DIGESTION AND ABSORPTION OF FATS

Fats require special digestive action before absorption because the end products must be carried in a water medium (blood and lymph) in which fats are not soluble. The enzyme LIPASE is the primary digestant used to split fats into fatty acids and glycerol. Although little actual fat digestion occurs in the stomach, gastric lipase does digest already emulsified fats such as in egg yolk and cream.

EMULSIFICATION is the real key to the proper digestion of fats. The large fat molecule presents comparatively small surfaces for the lipase to work on, so the process of emulsification by the action of bile produced by the liver is necessary. Bile breaks down the large fat molecule to tiny droplets which provide the lipase with an enormously increased surface to work on. This action takes place in the small intestine and the lipase involved here is a part of the pancreatic secretion.

The following diagram is very explicit as to the steps of fat digestion. We are aware that fat not needed for immediate use is stored in the body, but we must not lose sight of the fact that all stored fat did not come from our intake of fats. Much stored fat is formed from carbohydrates and as we mentioned previously, the body has a greater capacity to burn fats than it does carbohydrates. Thus, much of the fat ingested may be utilized and burned up by the body, while a percentage of the carbohydrate may be converted to storage fat.

DIAGRAM
OF FAT DIGESTION AND ABSORPTION

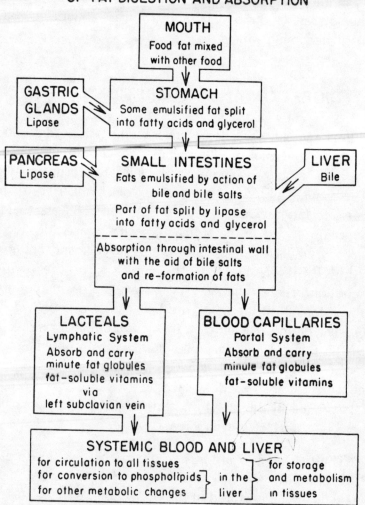

THE IMPORTANCE OF BILE

When a diet is low in protein or *high in refined carbo-hydrates,* little bile can be produced. If the amount of bile is insufficient or the gall bladder is not made to empty itself or the liver is not stimulated to produce bile, fats remain in such large particles that enzymes cannot combine readily with them; hence fat digestion is incomplete and fat absorption markedly reduced.

Part of the undigested fat quickly combines with any calcium and iron in the food to form insoluble soaps; thus these minerals are prevented from reaching the blood, and, the hard soaps, causing overly firm stools, bring about constipation. If this condition is prolonged, it can cause severe anemia, porous bones, spontaneous fractures and vertebral collapse.

Simultaneously, the lack of bile acids prevents the absorption of carotene and the vitamins A, D, E, and K plus the essential fatty acids. This can lead to a multiplicity of symptoms related to a deficiency of the vitamins (outlined later) or of the fatty acids.

It can thus be said that a complete digestive enzyme should contain bile salts and lipase as an insurance against the above. Also, those who have had their gall bladders removed may require bile salt supplementation the rest of their lives.

CHOLESTEROL

The mere mention of the word "cholesterol" is enough to strike terror into the hearts of many. It is probably as misunderstood a substance as any that appear normally in the body. Because few lay people know that cholesterol is extremely essential for body function — a constituent of

19

pituitary, adrenal, and gonadal hormones; converted to vitamin D upon exposure to ultraviolet light; acts as a conductor of nerve impulses — the fallacious theory that it was the major or sole cause of many heart problems was readily accepted.

The following facts can lead to a more rational approach to the whole cholesterol problem.

1. The less cholesterol you take in with your foods, the more your body produces.
2. The more cholesterol you take in with your foods, the less your body produces.
3. The atheromatous plaques found on the wall of the artery in atherosclerosis contain not only cholesterol, but fibrin, collagen protein, minerals, triglycerides and phospholipids plus other cementing cells which hold the whole thing together. Why was cholesterol singled out as the villain?
4. The atheromatous plaque, when it is first formed, contains no cholesterol at all. Fibrin (a protein in the blood needed for normal clotting) seems to be the first present. Is it possible that due to an inadequate dietary, the walls of the artery were getting weak and the fibrin stepped in to strengthen the arterial wall thus setting off a chain reaction causing other blood constituents to attach themselves?
5. The greatest rise in serum cholesterol occurs after the ingestion of excessive carbohydrates and not fat.

PREDICTION

I sincerely feel that we will shortly see butter, cheese, eggs and other cholesterol containing foods returned to their rightful place in the dietary of man. The restriction of these excellent foods in our diet is the most unscientific accepted theory in many years.

Carbohydrates

Carbohydrate foods make up from 50 to 70 per cent of the average American diet. There are probably several reasons for this; they are cheap, they produce energy very rapidly and they are very easy to digest. There are two basic forms of carbohydrates: soluble and insoluble.

SOLUBLE CARBOHYDRATES

The simplest and smallest carbohydrate molecules are the single sugars or MONOSACCHARIDES. They require no digestion and are readily absorbed from the intestine directly into the blood stream.

Glucose, also known as *dextrose,* is a monosaccharide and the form of carbohydrate to which all other forms are eventually converted for utilization by the tissues of the body.

Fructose, also known as *levulose,* is another monosaccharide which is commonly found in fruits and especially in honey.

Galactose, although not found in nature, is a monosaccharide derived from the breakdown of lactose, a disaccharide.

The double sugars or DISACCHARIDES are composed of three entities which may be broken down to simple sugars by action of specific enzymes either in the digestive tract or outside the body.

Sucrose, which is the common granulated or powdered white sugar or brown sugar, is one of the sweetest forms of sugar and also costs the least. Molasses, a by-product of sugar manufacture, is a crude form of sucrose and retains some minerals and vitamins from the original source which is usually cane or beet. "Raw Sugar" also falls into this general category, but contains less minerals and vitamins.

Maltose, also known as malt sugar, does not occur in nature but is manufactured by the body from starches by the action of the enzyme *diastase.* Of all the sugars, this one causes the least fermentation in the digestive tract.

Lactose, also known as milk sugar, is the least soluble of the disaccharides. It is also less sweet and is more slowly digested than the others. Lactose is an excellent medium for the growth of certain useful bacteria in the large intestines and has been used therapeutically following antibiotic therapy. There have been some claims that it enhances the absorption or utilization of calcium, but such a mechanism has not been substantiated.

INSOLUBLE CARBOHYDRATES

The insoluble carbohydrates are usually classified as starches, dextrins and cellulose. It is my opinion that cellulose does not fit into the general classification of food carbohydrates since the body cannot break it down and receive value from it. I have therefore made a complete separate classification under the heading Fiber which will immediately follow this discussion of carbohydrates.

Starches cannot be used readily by the body until the outer membrane is ruptured — either by grinding or cooking. The starch may then be acted upon by *ptyalin,* an enzyme contained in saliva. The starch is then changed into *dextrin* and finally into the double sugar, maltose. The enzyme, diastase, performs this function in the intestinal tract. We can thus see the importance of thorough mastication of foods, particularly those containing starches.

GLYCOGEN

Sugars which are not immediately used for the energy requirements of the body may be converted to glycogen which is then stored in the liver and muscles. It is this reserve which the body calls upon under stress conditions — the release of adrenaline initiates the immediate breakdown of glycogen into glucose. When the adrenaline is used up, the breakdown process stops and the construction of glycogen begins again. When the adrenals are sluggish, this process can be greatly retarded which explains to some extent the "wiped out" feeling that many with hypoadrenia complain of.

The only sugar which does not go through the glycogen cycle is glucose. All others are first converted to glycogen and then released after being changed to glucose as the body demands. This demand is partially due to the effect of adrenaline, as mentioned before, particularly on the glycogen stored in muscle tissue and also by the insulin from the pancreas. Adequate liver function is also all important for this delicate blood sugar balance, as it is in the liver that the conversion of the other sugars to glycogen and then back to glucose occurs.

CARBOHYDRATES TO FATS

Since the blood sugar mechanism is such a delicate mechanism and the overabundance of sugar can be of serious consequence, the body converts surplus carbohydrate into fat which is then stored as adipose tissue. AN OVERLIBERAL SUPPLY OF CARBOHYDRATE IN THE DIET IS THE CHIEF CAUSE OF OBESITY. In a diet lacking in carbohydrates, these stored fats are quickly converted back to sugars which are then used in the glucose-glycogen cycle. *this → adkins theory*

COMMENT

Carbohydrates are the most common and least important of all the foodstuff in our daily diet. The body is well able to convert fats and protein into glucose upon demand. Although many good foods contain carbohydrates, it is the almost totally nutritionally worthless foods that we condemn. The charts on the following pages list some of these "foodless" foods and equivalent sugar content.

"HIDDEN SUGARS" IN FOODS

FOOD ITEM	SIZE PORTION	APPROXIMATE SUGAR CONTENT IN TEASPOONFULS OF GRANULATED SUGAR
BEVERAGES		
COLA DRINKS	1 (6 oz. bottle or glass)	3½
CORDIALS	1 (¾ oz. glass)	1½
GINGER ALE	6 oz.	5
HI-BALL	1 (6 oz. glass)	2½
ORANGE-ADE	1 (8 oz. glass)	5
ROOT BEER	1 (10 oz. bottle)	4½
SEVEN-UP	1 (6 oz. bottle or glass	3¾
SODA POP	1 (8oz. bottle)	5
SWEET CIDER	1 cup	6
WHISKEY SOUR	1 (3 oz. glass)	1½
CAKES & COOKIES		
ANGEL FOOD	1 (4 oz. piece)	7
APPLE SAUCE CAKE	1 (4 oz. piece)	5½
BANANA CAKE	1 (2 oz. piece)	2
CHEESE CAKE	1 (4 oz. piece)	2
CHOCOLATE CAKE (Plain)	1 (4 oz. piece)	6
CHOCOLATE CAKE (Iced)	1 (4 oz. piece)	10
COFFEE CAKE	1 (4 oz. piece)	4½

FOOD ITEM	SIZE PORTION	APPROXIMATE SUGAR CONTENT IN TEASPOONFULS OF GRANULATED SUGAR
CUP CAKE (Iced)	1	6
FRUIT CAKE	1 (4 oz. piece)	5
JELLY-ROLL	1 (2 oz. piece)	2½
ORANGE CAKE	1 (4 oz. piece)	4
POUND CAKE	1 (4 oz. piece)	5
SPONGE CAKE	1 (4 oz. piece)	2
STRAWBERRY SHORTCAKE	1 serving	4
BROWNIES (Unfrosted)	1 (¾ oz.)	3
CHOCOLATE COOKIES	1	1½
FIG NEWTONS	1	5
GINGER SNAPS	1	3
MACAROONS	1	6
NUT COOKIES	1	1½
OATMEAL COOKIES	1	2
SUGAR COOKIES	1	1½
CHOCOLATE ECLAIR	1	7
CREAM PUFF	1	2
DONUT (Plain)	1	3
DONUT (Glazed)	1	6
SNAIL	1 (4 oz. piece)	4½

CANDIES

AVERAGE CHOCOLATE MILK BAR (example Hershey bar)	1 (1½ oz.)	2½
CHEWING GUM	1 stick	½
CHOCOLATE CREAM	1 piece	2
BUTTERSCOTCH CHEW	1 piece	1
CHOCOLATE MINTS	1 piece	2
FUDGE	1 oz. square	4½
GUM DROP	1	2
HARD CANDY	4 oz.	20

FOOD ITEM	SIZE PORTION	APPROXIMATE SUGAR CONTENT IN TEASPOONFULS OF GRANULATED SUGAR
LIFESAVERS	1	1/3
PEANUT BRITTLE	1 oz.	3½

CANNED FRUITS & JUICES

CANNED APRICOTS	4 halves and 1 Tbsp syrup	3½
CANNED FRUIT JUICES (Sweetened)	½ cup	2
CANNED PEACHES	2 halves and 1 Tbsp. syrup	3½
FRUIT SALAD	½ cup	3½
FRUIT SYRUP	2 Tbsp.	2½
STEWED FRUITS	½ cup	2

DAIRY PRODUCTS

ICE CREAM	1/3 pt. (3½ oz.)	3½
ICE CREAM BAR	1	1-7 depending on size
ICE CREAM CONE	1	3½
ICE CREAM SODA	1	5
ICE CREAM SUNDAE	1	7
MALTED MILK SHAKE	1 (10 oz. glass)	5

JAMS & JELLIES

APPLE BUTTER	1 Tbsp.	1
JELLY	1 Tbsp.	4-6
ORANGE MARMALADE	1 Tbsp.	4-6

26

FOOD ITEM	SIZE PORTION	APPROXIMATE SUGAR CONTENT IN TEASPOONFULS OF GRANULATED SUGAR
PEACH BUTTER	1 Tbsp.	1
STRAWBERRY JAM	1 Tbsp.	4

DESSERTS, MISCELLANEOUS

APPLE COBBLER	½ cup	3
BLUEBERRY COBBLER	½ cup	3
CUSTARD	½ cup	2
FRENCH PASTRY	1 (4 oz. piece)	5
JELLO	½ cup	4½

Dietary Fiber

Cellulose and hemicellulose are commonly listed as insoluble carbohydrates. They are the chief constituents of wood, of the stalks and leaves of all plants and of the outer coverings of seeds and cereals. Another fiber, lignin, commonly occurs in alfalfa but is not found in any abundance elsewhere. These substances act as the storage containers for water, starch, minerals and other substances for vegetation. Since their capacity to be digested is practically nil, these food factors have been relegated to a category of "lesser importance" in almost all nutritional books.

In light of recent in-depth studies on the importance of dietary fiber, it is my pleasure to offer you a category of foodstuff equally important, if not more so, than the recognized proteins, fats, and carbohydrates.

PANACEA?

The definition of panacea is: cure-all, universal remedy. The chemists of the world have diligently been seeking such a substance, but needless to say, always found only disappointment. If one is not careful, he may be accused of presenting such panacea when the true value of fiber is discussed. I will offer a few examples of the normalizing and preventive effects this substance exhibits.

DIVERTICULOSIS

The recognized cause of this disorder is excessive internal pressure on the wall of the colon, producing the characteristic "pouching" along the wall. When one of the pouches becomes obstructed with fecal matter and inflammation, infection and abscess formation can occur.

At this time it is called diverticulitis. The symptoms of diverticulosis are:

nausea	constipation	excessive gas
heartburn	bloating	abdominal pain

Although it is not considered possible to restore the structure of the ballooned-out portions of the colon to normal, over 88% of the patients treated with a high-fiber diet obtained dramatic relief from symptoms without recurrence — as long as the high fiber diet was maintained.

HEART ATTACKS

The common practice of villifying cholesterol in coronary occlusion and my objection to such have been outlined previously. There is, however, no question that a "clumping" of fats takes place during such an occlusion. The actual level of fat may be no higher than on any day previous, but at this particular time the fats seem to unite into a clot-like formation which is capable of stopping up some of the smaller arteries and arterioles. Up to this time the body had some means of preventing this dangerous coagulating of the fats normally in the blood stream (this would include cholesterol and all the other fats in the blood). Clinically there is evidence that the volatile fatty acids either have such an anti-coagulant effect or else synergize the production of such an agent. The breakdown of hemi-cellulose and cellulose by the intestinal bacterial flora produces these acids. Obviously in a diet lacking in dietary fiber, these acids would be absent.

Another fact giving rise to the "cholesterol theory" is the apparent high levels of cholesterol present in the blood stream in these heart patients. Consider this: One of the major functions of cholesterol is conversion by the liver into bile acids which are then normally eliminated in the feces.

On a low fiber diet the food remains in the colon for extensive periods of time with an explosive multiplication of putrefactive bacteria. These bacteria break down the waste bile acids into other substances including *lithocholate*. Lithocholate specifically acts back on the liver to cut down the conversion of cholesterol into bile salts — thus more cholesterol in the blood stream.

COMMENT:

A high-fiber diet produces the volatile fatty acids which have an anti-coagulant effect on the blood fats and also does not allow putrefactive bacteria, which depress bile acid formation from cholesterol, to build up in the colon.

HEMORRHOIDS, VARICOSE VEINS, AND PHLEBITIS

It is estimated that 50% of the population over the age of fifty suffers from hemorrhoids and an almost equal number are afflicted with varicose veins. Under most conditions, these two disorders are not emergency situations, but clots can form in either case and then serious problems can occur. With hemorrhoids, the distended vein usually becomes very tender and painful and can become ulcerated. A clot in a varicose vein produces the same symptoms plus inflammation due to the clot attaching itself to the wall of the blood vessel. It is then called thrombophlebitis. There is always the possibility that that clots can break loose and reach the lungs where a pulmonary embolism could occur.

How does dietary fiber concern these disorders? The small veins of the anus and rectum empty into the larger veins of the pelvis just as smaller rivers drain into larger ones. So do the veins of the legs which have an even harder task in fighting gravity to push the venous blood uphill into the large pelvic veins. But imagine the situation of a distended colon due to a low-fiber diet with dry, hard waste material collecting day after day. This distention produces pressure upon these drainage veins which creates back pressure on the smaller veins from 200 to 400 percent above normal. Is it any wonder that these blood vessels become swollen and engorged with blood? Adding to this constant pressure is the acute increase of pressure which comes from straining at stool. IT SEEMS ONE PROBLEM LEADS TO ANOTHER.

The addition of dietary fiber to the diet relieves the dry, hard condition of the stool and permits easy elimination. Thus, the physical pressure is removed from the venous drainage system and circulation is cleared in the entire area.

CANCER OF THE COLON

Every cancer researcher agrees that cancer can be caused by body surfaces coming in contact with potent cancer-causing chemicals known as carcinogens. Since the colon of the individual eating a low-fiber diet usually becomes sluggish with a time lapse of from two to ten days before expulsion, putrefactive bacteria abound. These putrefactive bacteria are not carcinogenic of themselves but let's look at what effect they have on otherwise harmless substances.

Bile acids are used to emulsify fats but are not absorbed into the body, they remain in the digestive tract to be eliminated with the feces. It is these acids which give the characteristic color to the stool. When these bile acids come in contact with putrefactive bacteria, two very powerful cancer-causing chemicals are produced: Apcholic

Acid and 3-Methyl-Cholanthrene. The implications of this is simple and unequivocal — AMERICANS WHO ARE ON LIFELONG LOW-FIBER DIETS ARE PROBABLY CONVERTING THEIR OWN HARMLESS BILE ACIDS INTO AWESOME CANCER-PRODUCING COMPOUNDS WITHIN THE CONFINES OF THEIR OWN LARGE INTESTINES.

COMMENT:

It is my fervent hope that everyone will accept fiber as the important food category that it really is. If one grasps the extreme importance of fiber in our diet, it can never again be consigned to a position of lesser consequence.

Enzymes and Nutrition

The subject of nutrition is intimately bound up with enzymes and their function in the body. Not only is digestion accomplished by the action of enzymes in the gastrointestinal tract, but the "burning" of food for energy and the chemical transformation of one material into another for use in the body are accomplished by enzyme reactions — a great many of them. We have previously observed that many individual enzymes will work properly only in the presence of certain cofactors, mineral ions and coenzymes, for example. Many coenzymes are composed, at least in part, of the essential nutritional factors we call vitamins.

WHAT ARE ENZYMES?

Enzymes are catalysts. Catalysts are agents that speed up a chemical reaction that otherwise would not take place or would take place so slowly as to appear not to be occurring. *Enzymes are made up of the amino acids found in protein* — another reason for quality protein in the diet. They are extremely intricate and complex in structure and act in very specific ways to accomplish their function, whether it be that of a molecular activator, a regulator or an overseer of a reaction.

WHICH ENZYMES SHOULD CONCERN US?

Quite obviously, all enzymes should be of concern to us, but many of them are extra or intercellular and other than a good protein diet, we have little control or influence upon them. On the other hand, the digestive enzymes can be enhanced by oral supplementation and are of primary importance to the student of nutrition. If it seems I am overemphasizing the fact that enzymes are made up in the body from proteins (amino acids) furnished by the blood stream, you are totally correct. A vicious circle occurs when either enzymes or protein are deficient — a lack of enzymes hinders the breakdown of protein and a lack of protein means that enzymes cannot be formed adequately or completely.

DIGESTIVE ENZYMES

Enzymes are specific in that each one acts only on a certain type of substances and brings about only one special chemical reaction. Thus when a digestive fluid has the ability to act on two or more kinds of foodstuffs, we know that there must be separate enzymes in it for the performance of each of these chemical reactions. Nor are the enzymes in different digestive juices that act on the same kind of foodstuff identical — we know this because they require different working conditions. The enzyme in the gastric juice that acts on protein requires quite a high degree of acidity to be effective, whereas there is a protein-splitting enzyme in the pancreatic juice that works well in either a slightly acid or even an alkaline medium.

Each of the digestive enzymes has some degree of acidity or alkalinity at which it works best and a certain range outside of which it will not work at all. A prominent example of this is the starch splitting enzyme in saliva (ptyalin) which acts only in neutral or slightly alkaline conditions such as found in the mouth and in the stomach before the food material is mixed with the acid gastric juice. As soon as the stomach contents become acid, the digestive activity of this enzyme is stopped.

In addition to optimum pH, two other conditions are required for the action of digestive enzymes. One is *surface contact* with the substance acted upon — for this reason intimate mixing of digestive juices with food particles which have been reduced to the smallest size possible or in an emulsified form (fats) presents the ideal circumstance for the enzymes to perform their function. The second condition is the removal of the end products formed by the reaction. Hence it is only in the small intestine, where the products of digestion are continuously removed by absorption, that conditions are favorable for digestive processes to run to completion. This in no way takes away the importance of the enzyme activity which begins in the mouth, continues in the stomach and is finally completed in the small intestine.

Digestion is actually quite efficient, there are normally two or more enzymes situated along the digestive tract for each type of foodstuff which passes by so that if one does not complete the job, the next one can take over. These enzymes are stimulated by a variety of factors:

1. Sight, smell or thought of food.
2. Chewing.
3. Hormones which are aroused by the presence of food in the upper tract.

Enzymes are inhibited by:
1. Fear, anger, worry.
2. Strong emotions.
3. Fatigue.

Hydrochloric acid and bile are both factors in digestion, but neither are enzymes. They do facilitate the work of the enzymes and are absolutely indispensable — hydrochloric acid for maintaining the acid media of the stomach contents so water soluble substances and proteins may be hydrolized and bile for the emulsification of fats so that the fat splitting enzymes have more surface to work on.

ABSORPTION

Absorption is the process by which the products of digestion pass through the lining of the intestine into the blood and lymph. (Note: Lymph is the intermediary between the blood and the tissues, since the blood is enclosed in blood vessels and does not come directly in contact with the tissue cells.) Simple sugars, amino acids, and short chain fatty acids are absorbed directly into the blood stream, but the products of fat digestion pass chiefly into the lymph, which is collected through tiny lymph vessels and finally emptied into the blood via the thoracic duct. Absorption takes place almost entirely in the small intestine with the muscular contractions of the intestine serving to bring the contents into close contact with the villi which contain both blood and lymph vessels.

ENZYME ACTION TABLE

AREA	FOOD CLASS	ENZYME ACTING	PRODUCT FORMED
Mouth	Starch	Ptyalin	Dextrins Maltose
Stomach	Proteins	Pepsin	Proteoses Peptones
	Casein	Rennin	Ca. Paracaseinate
	Pre-emulsified Fats	Gastric Lipase	Glycerol Fatty Acids
Intestine	Proteins	Trypsin	Polypeptides
	Proteoses	Chymotrypsin	Peptones
	Peptones Polypeptides Dipeptides	Erepsin	Amino Acids
	Fats	Steapsin	Simple Glycerides Fatty Acids Glycerol
	Starch Dextrins	Amylopsin	Maltose
	Maltose	Maltase	Glucose
	Sucrose	Sucrase	Glucose Fructose
	Lactose	Lactase	Glucose Galactose

Salivary Glands Secrete	Ptyalin
Stomach Glands Secrete	Pepsin and Hydrochloric Acid Rennin (childhood only) Gastric Lipase
Liver Secretes	Bile
Pancreas Secretes	Trypsin, Chymotrypsin, Steapsin, Amylopsin, Maltase, Erepsin
Intestinal Mucosa Secretes	Sucrase and Lactase

37

Chapter 2

STRESS

"I want out of this rat race! I can't stand the kids for one more day — I've got to get away! How can we pay the bills and still have money left over for groceries? If you don't relax, we're going to have to operate on that ulcer! These tension headaches are killing me."

Those are some of the familiar statements we hear every day from our associates, friends, and even family. All of them ar related to stress.

Stress comes in many different forms. We are all too familiar with what can be called emotional stress and the resultant nervous reactions that can occur. But stress may also be mechanical, physical, nutritional, chemical, as well as from radiation. In essence, stress can be considered anything that tends to inhibit self-will of the physical body and emotions, or to add something to the effort of the body needed to accomplish the above. Stress can be a passionate kiss as well as an obnoxious odor. As a result, there is some sort of common denominator to the body reaction to stress, no matter what kind is involved.

This common denominator can be summarized in Solyo'o analysis. Stress or pressure of some sort evokes a response from the body. It first is alarm. If the stress continues, the alarm turn to action or reaction. This is followed by rest or recovery so that the response is again available for the next stress. With age and continued stress, this rest period becomes longer and less efficient. This is the wear and tear period of stress reaction which turns into exhaustion or illness in the individual. Ultimately, when the stress reaction is totally exhausted, death ensues and there is neither stress nor reaction.

What we really are saying is that every response in the body creates some form of stress and, in a real sense, the way we respond to that stress is a measuring stick of our health.

INTERNAL STRESS REACTIONS

How this works internally is very interesting. There are three common reactions:
1. Inflammation and ulcer formation in the stomach.
2. The enlargement of lymph nodes.
3. Shrinking of the thymus gland.

The adrenal cortex glands control the bodily reactions to stress, usually with more cortisone secreted into the blood. When stress first contacts the person, the body over-reacts to be sure that a margin of success is guaranteed. Among these responses is the increased secretion of cortisone. As the stress continues, the body adapts to it and the secretion of cortisone is decreased or balanced against the stress. However, the amount secreted is more than normal so that the rest of the body adapts to this increased level of cortisone in the system. Among other reactions, the kidneys develop a slight vasoconstriction or tightening of the blood vessels which eventually leads to hypertension, one of the major killers in America today.

There are undoubtedly far more reasons for stress than we can ever cover in a book this size, but let's look at one that often is overlooked and therefore possibly more dangerous than others that are well known.

THE SUGAR STORY

Jane Doe was a thirty-five year old white female caucasian schizophrenic. Her main problem was that she would go into rages over some sort of trivial thing. Her behavior became so erratic that it was necessary to have her institutionalized for her own protection and that of her family. In the institution, her behavior patterns did not become more socially acceptable, in spite of heavy drug therapy, until someone noticed that her spells were apparently directly related to meals. Her behavior was notably worse after meals, particularly those that were high in processed carbohydrates. Approximately two hours after a meal, the rages reached their climax and gradually subsided over a period which could be several hours or more.

With this clinical picture in mind, her sugar metabolism was studied with a glucose tolerance test, which demonstrates blood glucose level changes. She was found to be hypoglycemic with the following curve: fasting 90, one-half hour 120, one hour 68, two hours 60, three hours 100, four hours 105, and five hours 98. Obviously something happened to her nervous control during the second half hour of this test which, incidentally, was the time that symptoms started.

Her diet was arranged so that she had no processed carbohydrates in the daily menu. The results were almost immediate, showing better emotional control, but not yet socially acceptable. The next step was to eliminate all natural carbohydrates in the form of fruits and some high value carbohydrate vegetables as well as grains. Now the results were quite satisfactory. She was absolutely normal so long as the offending processed and concentrated carbohydrates were not consumed. Deviations from this dietary pattern caused immediate emotional crises. It was later discovered that chemicalized foods also contributed to her clinical picture.

John Smith was a fifty-year old white male caucasian who suffered from a cardiac irregularity. His heart would race and become irregular on certain occasions when he exerted himself even to the slightest degree. It was not an incapacitating difficulty most of the time, but it certainly was an annoying experience. Having been interested in good nutrition for a number of years, he had already tried various suggestions. He had tried potassium, magnesium, B complex and other types of therapy all to no avail. For some reason he had never considered hypoglycemia as a possible cause of the condition until he obtained a glucose tolerance test from a friendly doctor. The results were very revealing. They were: fasting 88, one-half hour 117, one hour 140, two hours 130, three hours 120, four hours 90, five hours 50. An obvious hypoglycemic curve.

He was started on a routine high protein — high lipid diet and discovered that his heart irregularity was much less annoying though still present. Subsequently, when mega dosages of B complex, potassium, and magnesium were added into the program, the irregularity became a thing of the past.

Robert Jones was a 40-year old white male caucasian who was an announcer for a performance show where the traveling schedule was grueling with engagements in different towns, two or three times weekly. The precision of the performance was dependent, in part, upon his split second timing of the appropriate remarks on the P-A system. He had a marital problem wherein his wife was unhappy with the traveling situation. The eating patterns were less than good with much restaurant eating of the usual junk-type foods like hamburgers, french fries and cokes. He developed a very severe type of colitis wherein the bowels were almost constantly loose and, many times, the bowel was full of bright red blood. He and the family were quite concerned with the condition and he had consulted several of the country's major medical institutions. They all agreed that the condition was not a malignant state but that it was due to tension and the life style that he was living. He had many internal examinations and x-rays to prove this benign state. No satisfactory treatment was ever recommended. They were ready to resect or surgically remove his bowel.

His condition persisted and he ultimately had a glucose tolerance test performed. It showed: fasting 90, one-half hour 140, one hour 220, two hours 230, three hours 140, four hours 70, five hours 95. This curve, according to many orthodox physicians would be classified as a diabetic curve; but due to the drop to the low level in the fourth hour, it is in reality a diabetogenic type hypoglycemic curve. He suffers from the effects of hypoglycemia in spite of the fact that the glucose rises to high levels in the early hours of the test. He was immediately started on comfrey-pepsin (an herbal bowel soother and bulk producer) each hour, and given directions not to eat any processed carbohydrates like sugar and flour. He was also advised to avoid fruits for the first month of the treatment. The chronic bleeding stopped almost overnight. The colitis was under control within 72 hours and he had nothing but good reports following that, even though he still worked the same job with all its attendent pressures. The marital problem also settled down, since he felt more like a human being and could carry on a normal relationship.

All three of these case histories point to disturbed sugar metabolism leading to many of the signs of what we know today as stress. The logical question is then raised: "Is stress really another name for hypoglycemia?" Some might feel very comfortable in saying that this is true. I recall one physician saying to me: "It has been my experience that any symptom experienced by anyone is caused or aggravated by hypoglycemia until proven otherwise."

Since I tend to agree with such a statement, it is wise to

really understand how carbohydrates or sugars are used by the body.

CARBOHYDRATE METABOLISM

Carbohydrates may be classified in two ways, natural and processed. The processed are highly concentrated forms of glucose, while the natural are those found in foods like grains, fruits and vegetables. The natural can be either high concentrated or less concentrated. They are highly concentrated in certain fruits, vegetables, honey and grains. Both natural and processed forms of carbohydrates can be absorbed quickly into the blood to give high serum levels of sugar or glucose. When this happens, the pancreas "thinks" that the body is consuming a big meal, so it puts out an appropriate amount of insulin to do that job properly. The problem is that a big meal is not in the offing, resulting in a gross excess of insulin and a drastic lowering of the available blood sugar. It is this drop from a high glucose level to a low level which causes the physiology of the system to become upset.

Carbohydrates are used almost entirely in the system, particularly the nervous system (including the brain), for energy purposes only. When blood glucose levels fall, the nervouse system functions erratically with resultant symptoms as directed by your age, sex, occupation, et al. Symptoms produced in this manner include any symptom your body can experience but particularly: exhaustion, confusion, heart palpitations, diarrhea, gastrointestinal pain, back pains, and almost any other symptoms you can think of.

Glucose can be manufactured by the body from either fats or proteins; therefore, carbohydrates are not necessary in the diet for a balanced dietary. Certainly they are very tasty and more convenient for the body, but they are not an essential food. Actually, they are usually very rapidly absorbed into the blood, thus creating an undesirable situation. High protein — high lipid diets provide all the basic nutrients needed for metabolism and energy, both short term and long term. The body can be completely satisfied on a high protein — high natural lipid diet.

Unfortunately, the American diet is geared towards carbohydrate. True, it is also high in protein and fat because of the high meat intake, but the underlying high carbohydrate intake cannot be hidden. Here is a simple synopsis of factors leading to our present situation.

1. Since breast feeding has been a very unpopular practice in recent years, many infants are fed formulas of milk and sugar during the first year or more of life.
2. Solid foods for the infant are started at an early age with pureed fruits and vegetables that have been canned and processed with sugar and salt.
3. Rewards for good behavior include liberal quantities of candy and other sweets. Children's stories often proclaim the virtues of sugar: Little Red Riding Hood, The Gingerbread Man, etc.
4. Children, when weaned off the formula, are often put onto soft drinks, colas, non-colas and low calorie drinks. All have sugar or sugar substitutes which can often cause a reaction of the blood glucose identical to that seen when sugar is consumed.
5. Mid-afternoon snacks for growing children consist of various sweets like cookies and cola or kool aid.
6. Standards for breakfast are being set by TV commercials which toot the wares of devitalized cereals and drinks with added sugar.
7. Coffee with sugar is a common place beverage for children and teenagers as well as adults. Coffee is America's greatest addiction. Its reaction in the sys-

tem is to cause a rise in blood sugar even when consumed without added sugar.

8. The whole system in America is geared for the "coffee break" at 10, 2 and 4, just like Dr. Pepper suggests, because that is when blood sugar drops in most persons.

9. Convalescent diets in hospitals include coffee, toast with sugar and cinnamon, jello in liquid form and other high sugar products. Some hospitals even have mid-afternoon candy carts which bring patients "extra energy."

10. Bedtime snacks consist of something sweet with a bit of milk or a cola.

11. Nutritional support for the aged often includes more "high protein" jello (which contains more sugar than protein), white bread for easier digestion and always a dessert.

12. Cigarettes cause blood sugar to rise, each one as much as a spoonful of sugar. The adrenal cortices react against nicotine by extra utilization of vitamin C and raise the blood sugar by changing glycogen (storage sugar) into glucose as an assist in controlling the emergency caused by the nicotine.

13. Sugar consumption in the USA today consists of about 150 pounds per person per year. Incredibly, this figure roughly breaks down to mean the 60 teaspoonfuls of sugar are consumed daily by each one of us on the average. Some persons consume upwards of 150 to 200 or more teaspoonfuls of sugar daily.

14. Alcohol is closely related to sugar chemically and is metabolized like alcohol which connotes the evil nature of both.

All these and many more sugar laden characteristics of modern American life styles are the very cause of, or contribute to the cause of, America's poor health status.

SUMMARY

Many factors in the American life style work together to create a diet of carbohydrates. These are often called "food-less foods, empty calories," and a host of other names. In simple terms, they are deficient foods which do not furnish essential nutrients for the body. All fall short of actual bodily need so that when nutrients are stolen from other metabolic areas to effect their metabolism, gross deficiencies can result in the robbed areas. One universal argument used against this opinion is, "You mean to say a little bit of sugar in your wieners will hurt me?" The answer is: true, such a small amount will not cause trouble, but that is not the problem. Wieners are not the only sugar laden foods we consume each meal. Sugar is loaded into many foods. Read the labels. Coupled with the high sugar situation is the fact that even so called fresh vegetables, grains and fruits are often nutrient deficient since soils have been depleted by excessive agri-business techniques.

NERVES

A common description of an overreaction to stress is a 'nervous breakdown.' First of all, let us understand that nerves do not 'break down.' No one has ever seen a broken nerve — they just don't break. What does happen, in the presence of nutritional deficiency, is that the nervous system in the body begins to perform erratically and unresponsibly.

Of all the problems the human body is subject to, stress is one which is most responsive to proper nutrition. Sometimes we are so far in debt to our 'nutritional bank' that it is necessary to use supplemental food income or, more properly, intake to repay our loan and be even again. That is where concentrated food supplements come in handy.

As your nutritional pattern is approaching a break-even point, you will notice that your ability to accommodate stress becomes greater. The little things that used to irritate you so much no are no longer important. You will join that rank of privileged few who seem to thrive on stress. The reason is really quite simple — man was basically designed to withstand stress. We only need to read our history books to see that man has been under stress as far back as the records go.

Today we know what response is expected in the body from stress, what special nutrients are used by the body in accommodating to stress, and what to do if we are not accommodating. As far as the nerves are concerned, they are basically a protein structure, with generous amounts of fats as insulation and message carrier material. For normal nerve transmission, the B complex vitamin choline is very important, as is the mineral potassium.

We also cannot overlook the important role that glucose plays in this scene. The nerves use glucose as the fuel and if glucose aberrations exist, the nerve does not function properly. Hypoglycemia, a condition where the blood glucose levels fluctuate wildly, can possibly create such poor nerve transmission efficiency that the body begins to lose its ability to withstand even normal stress.

Since no one has had the courage to state that "stress is due to a lack of tranquilizers in the system," it should become readily obvious to everyone that these drugs are not the answer to the problem. But just as you repair or replace the roof when it leaks, so you should look to the building ingredients of your nervous system when it dysfunctions.

YOU AND STRESS

You are a person in society today and are confronted with stress. If it were not for stress, you would possibly not get out of bed in the morning. It is hunger or bodily necessities that make you mobilized each morning. Everything you do is based upon stress. Your body is geared to this, but when stress becomes excessive, problems begin to develop. According to Selye, stress evokes an alarm in the body. The body reacts to alarm according to the intensity of the stimulus and the training and control of the body. This is the simplest reaction to stress. As stress evokes repeated reactions, it eventually causes exhaustion. When stress continues on and on and recovery after rest becomes less and less effective, the adrenocortical glands become exhausted and disease develops. Ultimately there comes the one and only lifetime event, death. Death is the result of inability of the body to recover from stress. Death represents the ultimate in failure to recover while illness represents incomplete recovery. You have a unique reaction to stress based upon your anatomic and physiologic individuality. You are you, but you can change your body chemistry, which will change your response to stress.

SUGAR, NERVES AND YOU

Mr. and Mrs. Average America are victims of the system. They are conditioned to three meals per day of which breakfast may be missing or very light. Be it as it may on an individual basis, breakfast may consist of eggs, bacon and toast with butter, jelly and coffee with or without sugar or cream. There is usually a "coffee break" for more coffee and a sweet roll of some sort and a cigarette or two. Lunch consists of hamburger, french fries, ketsup, mustard, coffee or coke. One or two mid-afternoon snacks consist of some sort of sweet drink or coffee, cigarettes and maybe a candy bar or some other carbohydrate. Finally comes dinner, which is introduced by a cocktail of some sort, some nuts, corn chips, or munchies; then a salad, probably tossed with Roquefort dressing; a piece of meat, potato, vegetable, pudding or pie for dessert and coffee. This, with minor variation is the same sugar laden, empty calorie diet day in and day out for years on end. The body never becomes acclimated to this zig-zag, up and down available blood sugar situation. The "easily absorbed glucose" evokes a gross production of insulin because the pancreas "sees" a big meal coming along and acts accordingly. Only it is not a big meal, but just a little sugar so there is an excess of insulin available which causes the sugar levels in the blood to drop. This happens about each second hour every day. No wonder glucose metabolism becomes disturbed.

How your body reacts depends upon your particular individuality. Some, according to individual factors, react by having an ulcer. Others have heart attacks or become allergic. Remember, any symptom that can be experienced in the body can be caused or aggravated by blood sugar variations. You are unique in the anatomical and physiological natures of the body.

SYNOPSIS

1. Sugar and processed carbohydrates are vitamin and mineral deficient, which, when consumed by a person, makes the body deficient in a corresponding manner. Consuming one deficient food by itself may be unimportant, but it is not alone. So many of the convenience foods we consume today are heavily laden with sugar. When it's all added up, many consume the equivalent of 50 teaspoons of refined sugar daily. Such concentrated carbo-

hydrate foods must be eliminated and whole foods, preferably in the raw state should be substituted.

2. Nerve physiology, like systemic physiology, demands vitamins, minerals and enzymes to function correctly.
3. You are the product of your life-heredity, age, sex, occupation, etc. — and react to adverse stress; i.e. nutritional deficiencies in your own unique manner.
4. Correction of your problems that exist under present circumstances will require a change in life style, at least. It is your option, so do with it as you would. Here are some tried and true suggestions.

DISCUSSION

When the stressed problem person tries to build health patterns in his metabolism, two distinct factors must be considered. First, he is a person and needs all the various vitamins and minerals necessary for life just like any other person.

Secondly, because of his depleted state, he needs extra individual nutrients just to cause his metabolism to work correctly. He may have special inherent needs or just an intensified need because of his loss of nutritional integrity.

For example, the following formula represents the type of supplement which can act as an intensified normal intake substance upon which the more specific needs can be built.

SAMPLE FORMULA OF A BALANCED VITAMIN-MINERAL COMPLEX
USEFUL IN STRESS

Vitamin A	25,000IU	Para-Amino Benzoic Acid	100mg
Vitamin D	1,000IU	Calcium	750mg
Vitamin E	400IU	Phosphorus	150mg
Vitamin C	1,500mg	Iodine	225mcg

Vitamin B1	100mg	Iron	15mg
Vitamin B2	100mg	Magnesium	350mg
Vitamin B6	100mg	Copper	1mg
Vitamin B12	100mcg	Zinc	30mg
Niacinamide	150mg	Chromium	200mcg
Folic Acid	400mcg	Potassium	250mg
Pantothenic Acid	500mg	Manganese	30mg
Biotin	150mcg	Adrenal Substance	250mg
Choline	100mg	Selenium	200mg
Inositol	100mg		

In the stressed person, some special needs are obvious to the nutritional analyst. These include larger or mega doses of vitamin B complex. Actual dosages needed may be many times, even thousands of times, greater than RDA or MDR recommended levels.

Potassium may need to be taken in dosages that far exceed the usually accepted dosages, as is true with calcium and magnesium. A rule of thumb to follow is to keep taking larger and larger dosages if the apparent need still exists, so long as no ill effects are experienced. For instance, this could mean 200 — 400 mg of certain B complex vitamins if anticipated results are not forthcoming on lower dosages. No known toxic dosages for B complex are known. However, prudence and wisdom dictate proper amounts of all supplements used.

CONCLUSION

By careful management of the body, using diet, supplementation, enzymes, exercise and rest, one can improve the body's ability to cope with stress. It takes more than time and effort: IT TAKES PERSONAL DEDICATION AND PERSISTENT ENDEAVOR. Your health is a precious commodity. Once lost, it can only be regained with maximum effort. You cannot start yesterday; so at best, you must start today. Do something now to protect your health. It is your responsibility. No one else really cares as you should.

Chapter 3

THE MENOPAUSE

Menopause, often referred to as 'change of life' or 'climacteric'. is that transition period from reproductive function to one of a more enlarged vista of activity. Most women, by this time, have raised their children, gained the experience that a lifetime of trial and error has taught, and are now ready to depart on new avenues of enjoyment without 'that time' of the month to hinder activity.

Unfortunately, the woman who ceases to menstruate is often overwhelmed with physical and psychological phenomena which may make this time of life a miserable, tortuous experience. Since not all women go through this traumatic state, it obviously is not necessary — and I will attempt to outline in this booklet the reasons for the problems and the means to solve them.

WHAT REALLY HAPPENS?

The average age at which the menopause occurs varies from forty to fifty years of age, but the most common onset is from 45 to 48. There seems to be some relationship between the onset of puberty and the age at the time of menopause — girls who menstruate early often have a late menopause, late menstruation leads to early menopause. There is also a correlation between women who have had multiple children and a late menopause. Celibate women also seem to cease menstruating comparatively early.

At the end of the reproductive period, the ovaries gradually become inactive. This process is the reverse of changes that occurred at puberty, and a healthy woman on an adequate diet is as unaware of any disturbances as she was at adolescence. In some, the menstrual cycle ceases abruptly, in others irregularity sets in for as long as two years or more. As mentioned before, some women sail through this change of glandular function without any symptoms, but all too often some rather distressing activities take place.

The most common complaint is that of hot flushes, involving chiefly the face, neck, and often the upper part of the chest which becomes bright red, and there is a sensation of heat and suffocation. These vaso-motor events can occur as often as twenty times a day and many times at night, depriving the lady of necessary rest. Sweats may follow the flushes, or occur independently   at times so marked that the woman is drenched in perspiration requiring a complete change of clothes. She is often especially embarrassed when in a gathering of people, she constantly wants to open the windows while the others feel cool.

Other symptoms often observed are dizziness, headache, difficult breathing or shortness of breath, and palpitations of the heart which make the patient apprehensive and very uncomfortable. Mental depression is one of the most serious of the symptoms, leading to shaky marriage relationships and friendships. Although every doctor sympathizes with the menopausal woman, it is difficult to truly appreciate the multitude of physical and psychological changes which occur.

MISCONCEPTION

The psychological changes which are present such as

depression, anxiety, agitation, apprehension, inability to concentrate, etc., are often brought about by a misconception that this signals the end of a woman's attractiveness to the opposite sex. Many wives are sure that soon they will age, with wrinkling of the skin, lack of sex drive, sagging, flabby flesh and a host of other totally erroneous conceptions. With proper attention to diet, skin care and muscular tone, milady can look forward to a number of sexually active years (often more than her male counterpart) with more physical energy than she may have had when she was menstruating and losing a certain percentage of blood each month.

Yes, the ovaries have stopped producing estrogen, and everyone knows that estrogen is one of the essential hormones that give woman her feminine characteristics. But nature is not so hardhearted that she would disregard woman after her childbearing years have ended. In typical attention to detail, nature has set up a backup system in the adrenal glands which begin producing a hormone similar to estrogen when the ovaries cease functioning. This hormone performs all the functions of estrogen except that of preparing for conception. And herein lies the basis for most of the difficulties some women have with the menopause.

WHAT DOES ESTROGEN DO?

Estrogen is a broad term classifying several hormones secreted by the ovary which are responsible for the sexual growth and development which take place at and after puberty. They are essential for the development of secondary sex characteristics, such as body form and mammary glands; in the adult, they are essential to the normal functioning of the genital system. They are concerned with cyclic changes in the uterus, in particular those during the first half of the menstrual cycle.

In addition, estrogens bring about many other changes such as changes involving body form, condition of the skin, and mucous membranes, structure of the skeleton, water balance and various other metabolic activities. Some of the most important functions of the estrogens involve their relationship to other glands in the body by antagonizing or holding in check certain functions of other glands of internal secretion. Thus when ovarian control is removed, some of the other hormones act in relative excess. Incidentally this lack of ovarian function can come about normally during menopause or may be induced by surgery or irradiation.

THE PART THE ADRENALS PLAY

As I mentioned before, the adrenals are geared to take over the lack of estrogen by secreting a hormone which will perform all the functions of estrogen except produce the menstrual cycle. The only problem lies in an almost universal adrenal hypofunction. This state of affairs is best explained by the tremendous workload the adrenals have in our everyday life. They are the 'fight or flight' mechanism that comes into play with each and every stimulus we have from our external environment. They also are very involved in our internal well being; such things as blood sugar control are related to the adrenal secretions.

Now for a moment think about all the conditions or situations which irritated you this day. Let me list a few common ones.

1. Children wouldn't get out of bed in time for school.
2. Children wouldn't eat what was good for them.
3. Children didn't dress as you would like them to.
4. Worrying how you can pay the bills this month.
5. Saw on TV or read of a murder, kidnap, rape or other crime which really upset you.

6. Husband drove your car yesterday and didn't fill the gas tank up, leaving you with just enough to get to the service station.
7. The appointment you had at 10 o'clock is at least 30 minutes away by car and it is now 9:45.
8. You just heard that in eight years the Social Security reserves will be completely wiped out. It will be another seventeen years before you are eligible. What about all the money you put in?

I could literally go on and on, but the important point to be made is the constant stimulation which the adrenals are under. For each of the above hypothetical situations, the adrenals would have begun action to protect you from harm (and you must remember that most of these are in the form of psychological stress). Perhaps even greater is another factor of civilization which creates extra work for the adrenals.

A book was written called "Sugar — The Curse of Civilization." William Dufty, the newlywed husband of Gloria Swanson, has written an epoch colume with the title "Sugar Blues." Either or both of these books should be required reading for all students. They tell the story of how refined sugar creates a very abnormal situation in the body which constantly requires the adrenals to be called upon to secrete a hormone which is necessary to convert a storage sugar called glycogen into glucose for fuel. See Chapter on "Hypoglycemia" for further information on this.

All this only is valuable to the menopausal woman to demonstrate the possibility of adrenal sluggishness at the time in her life when she desperately needs quick and active adrenal function. As the ovaries cease to function, the adrenals should begin secreting a hormone which will replace estrogen in the hormonal balance of the body. If the adrenals produce only little or perhaps none of this hormone, then we have the typical symptoms of menopause. The already tired adrenal becomes more irritable and the following are the symptoms of adrenal irritability.

1. Dry mouth.
2. Circulatory imbalance — chills and flushing.
3. Temporary hypertension.
4. Internal nervousness and tremor.
5. Abnormal perspiration.

Do they sound familiar? Of course — they are the symptoms of the menopausal woman. The estrogen (or the adrenal hormone after menopause) normally acts to inhibit the sympathetic nervous system. Without this inhibiting action, the sympathetic nervous system allows all kinds of things to happen, such as blood which is normally pooled internally is suddenly rushed to the periphery which produces the hot flashes.

POTASSIUM AND VITAMIN E

It is interesting to note that potassium is a very important mineral for proper adrenal function and also for controlling our sodium balance. To be completely in balance we should take in twice as much potassium as sodium in our daily diet. From all evidence which has been gathered, just exactly the opposite is true in the average diet — twice as much sodium as potassium. When sodium is overabundant, potassium is excreted out of the cell and lost through excretory mechanisms. Thus we may get enough of this important mineral in our food but we have a sodium intake which is four times what it should be and the potassium is lost. Drugs such as sterioids and diuretics also force the excretion of this mineral. Because it is so necessary for glandular function, the menopause may be just the time for you to look to your potassium intake.

Another factor which should be considered is vitamin E. Although not reported in glowing headlines, medical literature is full of articles by reputable researchers who have found that vitamin E is the most practical and effective treatment for menopausal symptoms including hot flashes, high blood pressure, nervousness, heart palpitations, shortness of breath, insomnia, dizziness, fatigue and others. What is the possible mechanism which makes vitamin E the key in these instances?

One should consider the original work done on wheat germ oil which indicated that there was a sex hormone precursor available in this substance. During the menopause, when other enodocrine glands are taking over the hormonal function of the ovaries, does it not make sense that a little spark in the form of a hormone precursor might be of great value?

For this very reason, I always prefer a vitamin E which contains the raw wheat germ oil in addition to the tocopherols. Many times it is the unknown substances which make the difference between success and failure in a food supplement. Since some have a problem in handling oils, the addition of lecithin as an emulsifier can also be beneficial. As to amount, it has been estimated that the need for vitamin E during menopause soars from 10 to 50 times that of previous years. For this reason I suggest that a minimum of 600 IU of E be taken daily and if you can find a formula that contains both the wheat germ oil and lecithin you will have the greatest assurance of proper benefit.

STRESS PRODUCES
SPECIAL NUTRITIONAL NEEDS

From a great variety of experimental stress circumstances produced in animals we are capable to very specifically state what happens in the body when the additional stress of the menopause occurs in a woman. The nutritional needs will skyrocket, first in the particular needs of the pituitary gland which is the 'master' gland. Protein, vitamin E, the B complex vitamins are all necessary to maintain an adequate supply of pituitary hormone. Vitamin E, which is more concentrated in the pituitary gland than in any other part of the body, is thought to be particularly essential; it prevents both the pituitary and adrenal hormones from being destroyed by oxygen.

The adrenals are even more sensitive to dietary deprivation. A pantothenic acid deficiency causes the glands to shrivel and to become filled with blood and dead cells; cortisone and other hormones can no longer be produced and the many protective changes characteristic of the body's response to stress do not occur. Even a slight lack of pantothenic acid causes a marked decrease in the quantity of hormones released. The pituitary, adrenal, and sex hormones are all made from cholesterol, but without pantothenic acid, cholesterol cannot be replaced in the glands after once being used up. If generous amounts (up to 3,000 mg.) of pantothenic acid are given and the deficiency has not been prolonged and severe, the adrenal hormones can be produced normally within 24 hours.

We cannot overlook or underestimate the necessity of oils and butter in the diet. These are the sources of our sterols from which the hormones are made.

Although adrenal hormones can be produced without vitamin C, the need for this nutrient is tremendously increased by the menopause, and if under-supplied, the glands quickly hemorrhage and the output of hormones is markedly decreased. From experiments performed on guinea pigs, the need for vitamin C may be elevated 75 times over normal during menopause. Translated into human equivalents this means about 5,000 mg. daily of vitamin C.

HERBS ARE ALSO VALUABLE

The natives of many lands do not have the modern

laboratories to make drugs as we do and are forced to use nature as an assistant. Some of the herbs used through the ages for the menopause are.

Red Raspberry	Damiana
Cramp Bark	Squaw Vine
Sarsaparilla	Black Cohosh
Licorice	Ginseng

There appears to be specific action on the part of some of these in assisting the adrenals to produce hormones and others in acting as a general systemic tonic.

HOW ABOUT ESTROGEN THERAPY?

The advent of estrogen therapy was one of the greatest "symptom relief" therapies ever brought forth. Women on the brink of a nervous breakdown were miraculously brought back and became normal within a short time. I must impress on you however, that very few miracles exist today — and the ones that do are not in the form of a drug. Every miracle drug which has been discovered is fraught with danger, too often a danger which is not readily apparent. We now hear almost daily of the association of diseases with the use of estrogen therapy. Since estrogen has been used to induce cancer in rats, I would most sincerely recommend that one improve their dietary rather than resort to this method of alleviating symptoms. One doctor also stated that previously dormant cancer cells can be activated with the use of estrogen.

LOOK FOR A PROTEIN SHORTAGE

A common cause of hormone shortage is insufficient protein consumption. An experiment was reported wherein good nutrition was substituted for artificially administered hormones. Of the 726 patients on hormone therapy who were considered, 81 were vegetarians, and 56 of these were willing to accept temporary addition of meats to their diet. In the 56, estrogen levels, as well as other hormone levels, rose in 65 per cent when they began to eat meat. The vegetarians who refused meat were advised to cut down on cereals and cooked vegetables and concentrate on raw nuts and sunflower seeds. When one to four ounces of nuts or seeds were consumed by them daily, there was a rapid rise to good hormone levels. Pumpkin, squash and sunflower seeds were rated most effective.

A PERFECTLY NATURAL PROCESS

Menopause must be considered as a perfectly natural process. Although a shifting of gears is required, no drastic symptoms need occur as the adrenals take over the production of a hormone similar to estrogen, which has been produced by the ovaries for over 30 years. This sequence of events should proceed calmly and comfortably in a healthy, well-nourished woman.

The body is marvelously fitted with a system of glands — pituitary, adrenal, thyroid, etc. — intended to manufacture hormones whenever they are needed, and in the proper amounts. This they can be expected to do, if they are healthy and properly nourished. When hormone secretions are inadequate, the usually reliable glandular structure is probably ailing. There are effective measures for strengthening the glands:

1. Researchers have shown that glands respond to specific food supplements.
2. Since the cellular structure of the glands is controlled in its activity and ability to regenerate new cells, the

DNA or 'cellular blueprint' factor has been found to be of great assistance in rejuvenating an underactive gland. The DNA or 'nucleoprotein' as it is sometimes known, is the intelligence within a cell which rebuilds an identical cell when a worn out cell is dying. It forms RNA which is then sent out to the nutrient pool for specific nutrients such as amino acids, minerals, enzymes, etc., which are necessary to rebuild that specific cell. Dr. Harrower, in the late 1800s, first discovered that extracts of animal glandular material would help to restore human corresponding glands. Although DNA was not identified until 1960, Dr. Harrower and his work is still valid. Thus the use of pituitary, adrenal and other glandular extracts in assisting the body by the use of specific DNA factors to restore healthy function becomes a method of choice. These are available in tablet form in your local health food store.

SYNOPSIS

The following suggestions might be considered to avoid some of the 'change of life' difficulties so many women experience:

1. Many separate vitamins and minerals are suggested as being helpful by many doctors, but I sincerely believe that a good, high potency vitamin and mineral supplement will be more effective than any 'fragmented' approach. I have outlined a formula which you might use as a guideline when shopping.

MULTIPLE MEGA-POTENCY VITAMIN AND MINERAL SUPPLEMENT

Vitamin A .... 25,000 IU
Vitamin D .... 400 IU
Vitamin E .... 400 IU

Vitamin C	....	1,200 Mg
Vitamin B-1	....	60 Mg
Vitamin B-2	....	60 Mg
Vitamin B-6	....	60 Mg
Vitamin B-12	....	100 Mcg
Niacin	....	30 Mg
Niacinamide	....	30 Mg
Pantothenic Acid	....	100 Mg
PABA	....	60 Mg
Choline	....	60 Mg
Inositol	....	60 Mg
Folic Acid	....	400 Mcg
Biotin	....	100 Mcg
Calcium	....	1000 Mg
Magnesium	....	400 Mg
Phosphorus	....	150 Mg
Potassium	....	99 Mg
Iron	....	15 Mg
Iodine	....	225 Mcg
Copper	....	2 Mg
Chromium	....	500 Mcg
Manganese	....	15 Mg
Zinc	....	15 Mg
Selenium	....	20 Mcg

These are minimum quantities for a daily intake and some formulae may have added digestants, herbs and other food factors which enhance the product. Formulae such as the above are available from your health food store or vitamin supplier, so read your label and get the best.

2. If anything is used as an additional vitamin to the multiple, you should consider vitamin E because of the overwhelming evidence of its value. However, many find that the amount in the multiple is adequate. If you do decide on extra E, a formula containing wheat germ oil and lecithin will insure better utilization and results.

3. Herbs can be of amazing help in the menopause. The formula outlined previously has been used very effectively.

4. A proper dietary program of food selection with particular attention to proteins is a must. The Creative Restoration Diet outlined later in this book is a common sense approach to this problem.

5. The use of glandular extracts is also dramatic in the menopause. Again, I have outlined a complete formula of glandular extracts which support the entire endocrine system.

MULTIPLE NUCLEOPROTEIN FORMULA

Pituitary Extract	Thymus Extract
Adrenal Extract	Pancreas Extract
Heart Extract	Kidney Extract
Ovarian Extract	Ribonucleic Acid

By following the above, I feel that not only could menopausal symptoms be averted, but many presently suffering can be alleviated of much distress.

CHAPTER 4

ARTHRITIS

Arthritis is a kind of catch-all condition. Many complain of the symptoms, which are varied enough to cover many areas of the body. In general, the major symptoms are stiffness of joints; red, inflamed and swollen joints, muscular aches and pains; deformities of the hand and foot articulations particularly, and visible spurs on x-ray examination. Medically speaking, there are *no known specific causes* of this disease which afflicts a minimum of 25 to 30 million Americans. Some would like to blame past infections, bad teeth, injuries, etc., for the *chronic degenerative* disease we know as arthritis.

I have purposefully emphasized the fact that specific causes are not known in so-called scientific circles and the fact that arthritis is a chronic degenerative disease. I would like to tender some evidence that all chronic degenerative disease, and particularly arthritis, is due to an incomplete dietary intake of nourishing foods in as near their natural form as possible. We should understand that chronic degenerative disease is the slow, seemingly relentless, deterioration of the normal structure of the body. Medical science has produced wonderful measures to control emergency disease, but, by their own admission, seem powerless to halt the ravages of chronic disease.

Dr. Francis Pottenger, a well-known medical researcher, clearly established the relationship of a cooked food diet and arthritis in animals. He was able to produce arthritis at will, merely by feeding cats a diet of pasteurized whole milk.

Cats fed a diet of raw, whole milk had no evidence of arthritic disease whatsoever. This leads us to the obvious question: "Is the drinking of pasteurized milk the cause of arthritis?" The answer is not as simple as it may seem — I have personally found that a high percentage of arthritics are heavy consumers of pasteurized milk, ice cream, etc. But, I have also observed individuals with arthritis that used very little of these products. On the other hand, in every arthritic I have ever examined or interviewed, one factor stood out — they were consuming a great majority of their food in a cooked state and had a very limited intake of raw vegetables and fruits. Often the diet consists of meat, potatoes, salad, desserts, sandwiches, and processed cereals. Beverages are usually limited to coffee, tea, sugared soft drinks, and alcoholic beverages.

It has therefore been my conclusion, by whatever degree of scientific or unscientific logic you wish to assign, that when an individual uses a predominance of *uncooked* food in his diet, arthritis and other degenerative disease will not prevail in his body. I sincerely feel that the use of raw cream in the place of milk is a preventive factor, since the "Wulzen Factor" (also called the anti-stiffness factor) is only found in raw cream and many individuals who are not able to tolerate milk because of lactose intolerance are completely able to tolerate raw cream. By diluting with water, you have the ability to use it in any consistency you wish.

BUT I ALREADY HAVE . . .

All this sounds great, but what about if you already have arthritis? Several positive steps can be taken which will assist your body in normalizing its chemistry so further deterioration will halt, and normal repair processes be given a chance to restore normal function. It should be understood that these suggestions are not offered as a cure, but rather to assist the body in re-establishing normal function.

A. *You Must Cleanse The Body From The Toxic Buildup Which Overprocessed And Overcooked Foods Produce In The Body.* The Liver-Kidney-Bowel Cleansing Fast outlined later will accomplish this in short order. Many have remarked that the relief of pain is almost miraculous within just a few days.

B. *A Gradually Increased Program of Exercise On A Daily Basis Is A Must.* The exercise can consist of such simple activities as walking, swimming, bicycling, dancing, etc; or you can purchase a variety of home exercise units which are designed either for specific areas or for the general body. Some may find it more convenient to visit a health spa — but this is certainly optional.

C. *You Must Adhere To A Restorative, Rejuvenating Type Diet.* The Creative Restoration Diet which follows can be your guide to a pleasureful, healthy, and maximum variety type of eating pattern.

D. *Expose Your Face (without glasses) To The Sun At Least 15 Minutes Each Day.* This is in accordance with the work Dr. John Ott has done on the importance of full spectrum light entering the eye each and every day. This is not to advocate the direct staring at the sun, but just face the sun with eyes open for a minimum of 15 minutes each day. There have been reports of arthritic relief from just this simple mechanism, although our feeling is that it is just another link in the whole approach.

E. *Food Supplementation In Adequate Amounts To Help The Body In Its Restorative Function Has Proven Effective.*

1. Over 10 years ago Drs. E. C. Barton-Wright and W. A. Elliot, physicians at the Rheumatic Clinic in London, England, found that the symptoms of *both* osteo and rheumatoid arthritis were relieved by the use of oral

Pantothenic Acid, one of the B Complex vitamins. According to Dr. Barton-Wright, arthritis is caused, at least in part, by insufficient intake of pantothenic acid. He attributes such an insufficient intake to the highly processed food diets so common in the western world.

2. Dr. John M. Ellis, Chief of Medical Staff at Titus County Memorial Hospital, Mt. Pleasant, Texas, has studied another of the B Vitamins since 1961. His work on Vitamin B-6 (Pyridoxine) is thoroughly and completely reported in two books which he has written, "The Doctor Who Looked At Hands," and "Vitamin B-6: The Doctor's Report." His conclusions regarding the role of B-6 in arthritis were as follows: decreased finger pain, stiffness and numbness relieved, reduced pain in the shoulder, hip and knee areas, and a cessation of nighttime muscle cramps. The amount of Vitamin B-6 used varied, but the average dose was from 50 to 100 Mg. daily.

3. Dr. Roger J. Williams, the distinguished biochemist who is perhaps responsible for more original work in the field of vitamin research than any living scientist, points out the relationship of Vitamin C, Vitamin A, Vitamin B-2 (Riboflavin), the minerals Calcium and Magnesium to arthritis, since it is a 'Collagen Disease.' Collagen is the elastic protein substance which makes up cartilage — which is the cushion material around the joints of the body. Cartilage is subjected to a lot of abuse just from normal motion of the body and requires continual rebuilding to do its job of absorbing the jolts and strains that would destroy bone surfaces, if they were not protected by the cartilage. The above nutrients play an important part in the normal formation of replacement collagen which makes up a great portion of cartilage — therefore a lack of any one or a deficiency of all of them would impede cartilage cell repair and open the door to arthritic symptoms.

4. We really should bring the drug, cortisone, into this

discussion, since the relief which some obtain from its administration is almost miraculous — but temporary and loaded with side effects. Just what does cortisone do? The adrenal glands are one of the most important glands we have in the body when we are dealing with stress — and arthritis is certainly a stress disease. The adrenals produce many hormones which are needed to 'trigger' functions in the body. One of those functions is that of rebuilding and maintaining healthy cartilage and connective tissue. Interestingly enough, Pantothenic Acid, vitamin C, and the mineral Potassium are all involved in the normal production of these adrenal hormones, including cortisone. We stress that other hormones produced by the adrenals are needed to work in harmony with cortisone for normal function, thus the use of cortisone alone produces a hormonal imbalance with all kinds of side effects. On the other hand, the restoring of the above mentioned nutrients to the dietary intake of an individual will enhance the normal production of all the adrenal hormones. So, an absence of any of these vital nutrients could cause poor cartilage repair which in turn would lead to arthritis.

5. The use of 'folk remedies' should also be brought into this discussion. Through trial and error, often by accident and without knowing the chemistry behind the effect, some of the most dramatic advances in medicine have been made by lay persons. A favorite remedy for years has been equal parts of cream of tartar and epsom salts in a glass of water morning and night. When we look at the components of these two common ingredients, we can see why there was a certain degree of success in their use. Cream of tartar is made up largely of potassium and epsom salts is primarily magnesium — both of these minerals have been discussed previously in their relationship to the health of the adrenal glands and the utilization of calcium.

One of the most difficult 'folk remedy' for me to

determine the mechanism by which it was effective was the use of "Certo", a product used by homemakers in the preparation of jams and jellies. It is composed primarily of fruit pectin, and until I learned that many arthritics have an extraordinary amount of lead in the blood stream, the answer evaded me. Lead replaces calcium in the bone structure, which leads to all kinds of calcium related disorders. Pectin renders it insoluble in the body, and so I had my answer. The reason these remedies are sometimes ineffective is that the mechanism by which they work for some may not be the cause of the problem with others. Again, we must emphasize a total approach, only then can we have some assurance of success in the different types of arthritis.

A TRUE LINK

What this research indicates is that there is a true link between a 'chronic degenerative disease' such as arthritis and adequate availability of nutrients. I would like to quote from Dr. Roger J. Williams book, "Nutrition Against Disease: Environmental Prevention." *While medical education has put a damper on experiments in which the nutrition of arthritics might have been studied and manipulated in an expert fashion, there is excellent reason for thinking that if this were done, sufferers could get real rather than palliative relief. There is even a good possibility that individual arthritics will be able — if they are lucky and make intelligent trials — to hit upon particular nutrients or nutrient combinations which will bring benefit.*

"I certainly would not want to give the impression that the management of these diseases is simple. But I do affirm the dictum that nutrition should be tried first. On the basis of reports presently available, the items that certainly need to be considered are niacinamide, pantothenic acid,

riboflavin, vitamin A, vitamin C, vitamin B-6, magnesium, calcium, phosphorus and other minerals. The objective is to feed adequately the cells that are involved in keeping the bones, joints, and muscles in healthy condition."

I don't think it could be said more clearly. Only one cautionary word — do not use fragmented nutritional supplements. Find a formula that contains all the nutrients and use that as your foundation product. If after you have used it for some time, you find there is an additional need for some nutrient — vitamin C as an example — add it to your program. Remember that all these substances work as a team and the total effect of all is far greater than individual effects.

Here is an example of what I would consider to be a complete food supplement with emphasis on the nutrients which researchers have found of assistance in arthritis:

Vitamin A	25,000 IU
Vitamin D	400 IU
Vitamin B1	50 Mg
Vitamin B2	50 Mg
Vitamin B6	100 Mg
Vitamin B12	500Mcg
Vitamin C	1500 Mg
Vitamin E	400 IU
Niacin	50 Mg
Folic Acid	400Mcg
Biotin	25Mcg
Pantothenic Acid	1500 Mg
Choline	50 Mg
Inositol	50 Mg
Para Amino Benzoic Acid	50 Mg
Glutamic Acid HCl (Glutamic)	100 Mg
Bromelain	100 Mg
Citrus Pectin	150 Mg
Lemon Bioflavonoids	100 Mg
Calcium	1000 Mg
Magnesium	400 Mg
Iron	15 Mg
Iodine	225Mcg

```
Manganese  ...................  25 Mg
Potassium  ...................  99 Mg
Chromium  ..................  500Mcg
Zinc  ........................  10 Mg
Copper  ......................  5 Mg
```

TRY THIS RESTORATIVE, REJUVENATING PRO-
GRAM AND BE BLESSED TWO TIMES: FIRST WHEN
YOU FIND THAT YOU CAN CONTROL AND DIS-
CIPLINE YOUR BODY AND SECONDLY WHEN THE
FREEDOM FROM PAIN AND INCONVENIENCE OF
DISEASE IS RESTORED TO YOU. REMEMBER THAT
SELF-DISCIPLINE IS LESS LIMITING THAN DISEASE IS.

Chapter 5

HYPOGLYCEMIA

HYPOGLYCEMIA & HYPOADRENOCORTICISM

The two terms above mean different things, but for all practical purposes are synonymous. Hypoglycemia means low blood sugar, and hypoadrenocorticism means low functioning of the adrenal glands. Seldom heard of just a few years ago, today more and more physicians are finding that many of the patients that were real problems are actually hypoglycemic. It only takes a minute to look at the myriad of symptoms to understand why this disorder can be masked and misdiagnosed.

Headaches	Overactive child
Sudden fatigue	Behavioral problems
Irritability	Seizures
Insomnia	Convulsions
Forgetfulness	Asthma
Anxiety	Hay Fever
Depression	Eczema
Crying Spells	Hives
Feeling of faintness	Sinusitis
Sudden hunger	Reduced sex drive

Exhaustion	Stomach pain
Inability to concentrate	Digestive disorders
Dizziness	Colitis
Cold Sweats	Diarrhea
Feeling shaky	Fearfulness
Edema	Blurred vision
Dry mouth	Shortness of breath
Twitching of eyelids	Cold extremities

Craving for sweets, alcohol, coffee, coke. Eating sweets or smoking will temporarily relieve symptoms.

After reading that list of symptoms, one could say: "But that just about covers everybody." The unfortunate situation is that a tremendous number of people are hypoglycemic and never know it. They mask the symptoms by excessive eating of sweets, drinking alcohol, consuming large amounts of coffee, or smoking continually. Others are being treated for ulcers, gastritis, 'nerves,' mental problems, heart disease, and any number of other 'misdiagnoses.'

WHAT IS IT

The condition of hypoglycemia or hypoadrenocorticism, can be complex to understand if all the involved mechanisms in the body are detailed. For purposes of easy comprehension, we shall use an 'overview' to explain what occurs. The body is really not set up to handle concentrated sugars — which too often make up a large part of our diets. Although sugar is the fuel on which our entire body runs, the use of a concentrated form such as pastries, pies, sugar coated cereals, candy, etc. overloads the delicate control mechanism and the pancreas overreacts by producing too much insulin, which in turn burns up or converts too much sugar. Now the body will again cry out for food and too often a wrong choice is made when this need is acute. Thus a vicious circle is established with side effects of malnutrition and all the attendant symptoms resulting from it. The malnutrition occurs because too little protein rich foods and vitamin and mineral containing vegetables and fruits are used. Instead, the convenience type foods take over a large percentage of the daily intake — and these are notorious for having nutrients processed out, or even non-existent to begin with. They are, in fact, often called 'junk' foods.

The sugar which the body cannot use as energy when it has been acted upon by insulin will be converted to glycogen, which is the 'instant reserve fuel' for the body, and is stored in the liver and muscles; or what cannot be stored as glycogen will be converted to fat. This can be one of the major causes of uncontrollable weight gain for certain individuals.

CONVERSION MECHANISM

In normal body function, there is a conversion mechanism, which protects us against the rapid drop in blood sugar such as in the aforementioned situation. The adrenal glands, which are the stress response glands, secrete a hormone which begins the change process of glycogen back to sugar. This same response is brought into play when fear, anger, or emergency situations call for great strength. Such an expenditure of energy requires lots of fuel, so glycogen from the liver and muscles is immediately turned into sugar.

Taking this process one step further, the body replaces the glycogen reserve by converting adipose tissue (fat) into glycogen, in order to keep a ready reserve.

The important thing to remember is that all these mechanisms are dependent upon hormones, and particularly upon adrenal hormones. Recent research indicates that the single most common cause of hypoglycemia is a poorly functioning adrenal system. Sluggish adrenals can cause a slow conversion of glycogen to sugar in time of need, and if that occurs the craving for something sweet becomes overpowering.

HYPOGLYCEMIC SINCE BIRTH

Many infants are born with adrenal glands which function poorly because the mother had an adrenal problem. She may have had this problem for a long time, or may have been under considerable stress during pregnancy, or may have eaten a typical American diet high in refined carbohydrates and low in protein. The infant then, in many cases, starts out in life with colic, diaper rash, respiratory disorders, and various adverse reactions to formulas. Formulas are too often given that are high in carbohydrates, which merely add to the innocent child's problem.

HYPOGLYCEMIC PROGRESSION

Assuming that you were not born hypoglycemic, what causes some to become victims of this disorder and others escape? The mechanism of hypoglycemia goes something like this:

1. Excessive intake of refined carbohydrates.
2. Rapid rise in blood sugar with resultant excess production of insulin.
3. Rapid decline in blood sugar because of the excess insulin — below normal blood sugar.
4. Adrenal response to convert glycogen to sugar for emergency.

5. Repeat above pattern many times a day.
6. Adrenals get tired — don't respond as quickly.
7. Emergency! Body in danger of fainting, need sugar fast!
8. Person eats or drinks a high sugar containing product.
9. Blood sugar rises rapidly and cycle starts all over again.

Following such a progression, it is not difficult to see why a hypoglycemic becomes a physical and emotional yo-yo. When the blood sugar is elevated, they are feeling fine, when it drops, they have all kinds of symptoms.

OTHER STRESS FACTORS

There are many kinds of stress in our environment, and they all directly affect our adrenal glands, since they are the stress glands. Some examples are: infection, pain, over-exertion, child bearing, burns, fractures, business problems, domestic disagreements, and drugs. Prolonged stress has a degrading effect on the body, particularly the adrenals, and eventually, reduced efficiency to cope with stress ensues. Since the adrenals play such an important role in the hypoglycemic situation, such stress can bring on the condition or make it worse if it already exists.

Another factor which enters into this picture is the ability of an individual to 'whip' his adrenal glands into functioning by the use of a variety of stimulant drugs. The two most common are coffee and tobacco. Both of these products are addictive because of their action on the adrenal gland. The stimulation of the adrenal synergizes the glycogen conversion mechanism and temporary rise in blood sugar gives the individual a 'lift.' It doesn't take much programming of the body to automatically reach for a cup of coffee or a cigarette when you are feeling 'down.' In order to overcome his condition, the hypoglycemic must make up his mind to stop both these drugs totally.

DIAGNOSIS

Although it is not used as often as perhaps it should be, the test for hypoglycemia is fairly simple. Approximately 100 grams of glucose (sugar) is administered after a fast of at least 12 hours. A blood sample is taken before the sugar is taken and again each hour for a period of 5 or 6 hours. The deviations above and below the fasting level are diagnostic, particularly below. Many individuals find that they feel faint or may even lose consciousness at the second or third hour, because of the extreme drop in blood sugar levels.

It should be taken into consideration that the circumstances of this test are not those of everyday life. It is possible for the borderline hypoglycemic to show a fairly normal blood sugar curve in the laboratory, while under the stress of his job or other factors, may actually be hypoglycemic due to the added strain on his adrenal glands, which then respond sluggishly to the demand for glycogen conversion.

DON'T FORGET THE LIVER

We have been talking a great deal about the adrenal glands and their importance in dealing with the problems of hypoglycemia. Another organ in the body which plays a great part in the blood sugar regulation is the liver. Since it is in the liver that sugar is converted to glycogen for storage, then stored in the liver as well as muscle tissue, and, as needed, converted back to sugar again, it is easy to see the importance of good liver function for proper blood sugar levels.

The liver can be damaged or have its functional capacity

reduced by several factors: excess alcohol consumption, tobacco, smog, infections, and toxic drugs. Fortunately, the liver is one of the fastest regenerating organs in the body (demonstrating its importance) and, once these liver damaging factors are overcome, it will restore itself and carry out the many body functions it performs.

I highly recommend the Liver-Kidney-Bowel Cleansing Fast outlined later in this book for those who feel that this could be a problem or complication in their search for optimum health. The opinion exists in the minds of some that hypoglycemics are not supposed to go on fasts. I would like to point out one fact: In most cases the hypoglycemia is triggered by the ingestion of a high carbohydrate food. In the Liver-Kidney-Bowel Fast, no sugar is contained other than what might be naturally present in the lemon juice and this will be so diluted that no emergency signal is sent to the pancreas for excess insulin. Thus, most hypoglycemics will reap nothing but benefits from the use of this fast.

HYPERINSULINISM

Hyperinsulinism is another term that some use practically synonymously with hypoglycemia. Literally interpreted, the term means an excess amount of insulin. We have seen how this occurs in the progression of this disorder. Another interesting tie-in of the adrenal glands and the pancreas is seen here. When the amount of insulin necessary to do the job on a given amount of sugar has been secreted, it is the job of an adrenal hormone to send a message to the pancreas to stop producing insulin. A sluggish adrenal will be late in this function, thus allowing an overproduction of insulin with a resultant excessive lowering of the blood sugar.

DISASTER

"I'm just so tired all the time." "I don't seem to have any pep." "What makes me so nervous?" "I think I'm going crazy." I'm always depressed, even when things are ok." "I've tried every medication and doctor around, but they can't find out what's wrong with me."

The above comments are constantly heard, not only by doctors, but by lay people as well. Hypoglycemia can often be the condition that seems to evade the diagnostician, because until recently, it was not considered a serious possibility or disease. Many doctors were wont to tell their patients with the disorder to carry candy or sugar lumps on their person at all times and take one when the symptoms arose. Unwittingly, they were increasing the severity of the disorder by their advice!

Various authorities have estimated that up to 100 million persons in the United States suffer from this condition. Such a high incidence of hypoglycemia (almost 1 out of 2) may be a significant factor contributing to our country's woes, since hypoglycemics are not always operating at their highest potential; consequently they can cause problems for themselves and for others. During the times when their blood sugar is low, their working efficiency can be drastically reduced, they can also be involved in needless arguments because of their hyperirritability, and also can have many severe mental and physical problems.

RESTORATION PROGRAM

Now that we are familiar with hypoglycemia, its symptoms, causes, and effects, it is time we thought about doing constructive restoration to the body. It is only with such a program that the relentless, debilitating of the human body by a disorder such as hypoglycemia can be overcome. Many have said to me, "I don't know if I have hypoglycemia and I don't have the money for the tests and doctors." My answer is simple — try the program and if you feel better, stay on it! At the very worst, you are following a good diet and you body will benefit from it.

Step One: Cleanse your body and particularly your liver by going on the Liver-Kidney-Bowel Cleansing Fast outlined later. It can and has performed miracles for many; you are no exception. Over and above the obvious detoxification that occurs, mental clarity can be achieved beyond any other method.

Step Two: Follow the Carbohydrate Intolerant Diet Program very closely. On such a program you can expect to see changes in just days.   (Outlined later in book).

Step Three: Rebuild the glandular structure in your body, particularly the adrenals. We now know that DNA concentrates in combination with RNA can have a tremendous rejuvenating effect on target glands. It is my opinion that very seldom is just one of the glands involved, so we suggest the use of a tablet containing adrenal, pancreas, pituitary, and other glandular factors as the best approach.

Step Four: Because of the high carbohydrate diet which the hypoglycemic has been using, there are some rather severe nutritional deficiencies present. The use of a very complete high potency vitamin and mineral support is an absolute must for best and quickest results. Such a product should contain all the B Complex in balanced form, at least 400 IU of Vitamin E, 1200 Mg. of Vitamin C, all the minerals, but especially Potassium, Chromium, and Zinc. This can be purchased in one formula from your health food store.

SAMPLE FORMULA OF A BALANCED VITAMIN-COMPLEX

Vitamin A	25,000IU	Para-Amino Benzoic Acid	100mg
Vitamin D	1,000IU	Calcium	750mg
Vitamin E	400IU	Phosphorus	150mg
Vitamin C	1,500mg	Iodine	225mcg
Vitamin B1	100mg	Iron	15mg
Vitamin B2	100mg	Magnesium	350mg
Vitamin B6	100mg	Copper	1mg
Vitamin B12	100mcg	Zinc	30mg
Niacinamide	150mg	Chromium	200mcg
Folic Acid	400mcg	Potassium	250mg
Pantothenic Acid	500mg	Manganese	300mg
Biotin	150mcg	Adrenal Substance	250mg
Choline	100mg	Selenium	200mg
Inositol	100mg		

MULTI-GLAND FORMULA

FEMALE

Ovarian Substance	60mg
Whole Pituitary Substance	20mg
Adrenal Substance	60mg
Thymus Substance	60mg
Pancreas Substance	60mg
Kidney Substance	60mg
Heart Substance	60mg
Ribonucleic Acid (RNA)	60mg

MALE

Prostate Substance	60mg
Whole Pituitary Substance	20mg
Adrenal Substance	60mg
Thymus Substance	60mg
Pancreas Substance	60mg
Kidney Substance	60mg
Heart Substance	60mg
Ribonucleic Acid (RNA)	60mg

BLOOD SUGAR CURVES

Many ask what the glucose tolerance test tells the doctor. In a very simplified form, the following charts show some of the typical graphs that result from such a test. Although the degree of blood sugar drop is not always paralleled by the severity of the symptoms, it is a good indicator. Some individuals also react under stress conditions with a drastic drop in blood sugar levels, while under normal conditions their blood sugar levels are comparatively normal. This type of condition is the most difficult to diagnose. My suggestion to an individual who has hypoglycemia type symptoms, but has been told he or she is not hypoglycemic, is to go on the hypoglycemic program. Nothing can be lost and the benefit can be immediate.

COMPARATIVELY NORMAL BLOOD SUGAR CURVE

X. The fasting blood sugar level and the time when a measured amount of glucose is administered.

Y. Base line or percent of blood sugar below which is considered low blood sugar.

CRITERIA:

1. 6-hour reading should be within 5% of fasting level.
2. No point should fall below the base line.
3. The 1-hour level must rise at least 50% above the fasting level.

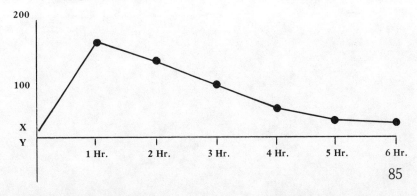

85

HYPOGLYCEMIC BLOOD SUGAR CURVE

Note: this is only a relative comparison, there are severe cases where at the 3-hour level the blood sugar level is already below the base line.

On the other hand, there are pre-hypoglycemics or "stress" hypoglycemics who have a 1 or 2% dip below the base line at the 5th or 6th hour under test conditions. But, under the daily stress of living, this may drop 10 or 20% below the base line and all the attendant emotional and physical symptoms appear. Thus the interpretation of 'borderline' or 'almost normal' is rather dangerous to the patient because he may then consider his problems in the realm of 'mental' and use tranquilizers, coffee, cigarettes, candy, or alcohol to cover up the symptoms.

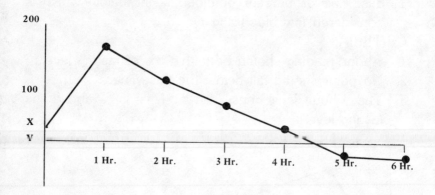

DIABETIC BLOOD SUGAR CURVE

Note initial high fasting blood sugar level which does not return after glucose intake even to that elevated level but remains high after six hours.

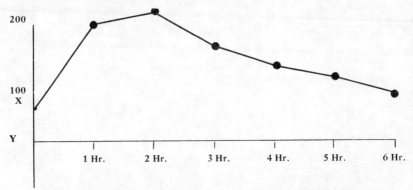

DIABETIC-HYPOGLYCEMIC BLOOD SUGAR CURVE

A simple 2 or 3-hour glucose tolerance test on the above individual would convince any physician that the patient is a diabetic. The fact is that he is both diabetic and hypoglycemic at this point and a hypoglycemic diet will solve both problems while an insulin program would create even more serious hypoglycemic symptoms. Also the patient will have chronic difficulty regulating the insulin intake. It is this type of patient that really points out the need for a full 6-hour glucose tolerance evaluation.

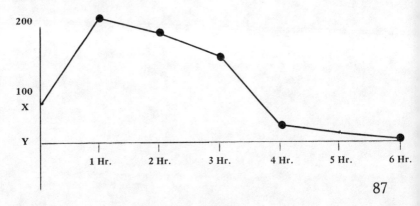

Chapter 6

THE OVERWEIGHT PROBLEM

There is probably no condition of the human mechanism that has received as much attention from the press as the overweight problem. The favorite headline of many magazines is "New Weight Loss Diet — Quick and Easy." It has been said that there are more weight loss diets around than successful users of such diets.

There can be no doubt that even with the plethora of diets available, overweight is still one of the most prevalent physical conditions which individuals would like to correct. There have been some rather successful programs — The Atkins Diet (high protein, medium fat, low carbohydrate intake), Weight Watchers (proportioned foods with a psychological incentive via group testimonial meetings), TOPS (Take Off Pounds Sensibly) — similar to Weight Watchers, etc. The problem with these programs, as I see it, is that there is an improper emphasis on food intake. On the Atkins diet, the high protein diet becomes very monotonous, particularly after a certain amount of weight has been lost. The weighing of food portions also becomes a tedious task and is difficult to accomplish under many daily circumstances.

It will be my contention that once you understand the mechanism of weight gain, you can then rather simply control your weight at will — but without the severe restrictions and/or the possibility of doing bodily harm because of an imbalanced diet.

HOW THE BODY ACCUMULATES FAT

Although many mechanisms are involved, the body basically accumulates weight when the total energy factor assimilated from the food eaten, exceeds the amount of energy expended in daily living. This can have both nothing and everything to do with your food intake. Let me explain: When the food intake is high in carbohydrates, which are very readily and rapidly absorbed from the intestinal tract, a rapid rise occurs in the blood sugar. Insulin is then poured into the blood stream from the pancreas to assist in the conversion of that form of sugar to glucose, which is the type of sugar the body literally burns for fuel to furnish energy. An excess of this substance, commonly called sugar, can lead to very serious problems, so the body has a built-in defense mechanism to control it. The carbohydrate (sugar) which is in excess at that particular time is converted to glycogen which can be stored by liver and muscle tissue. Then, when the body has an immediate need for energy, this substance is converted to glucose. But often there is an excess which the storage mechanism in the liver and muscle cannot handle. This excess is then converted to fat which then elevates the blood fat level (including cholesterol and triglycerides) and eventually is deposited as adipose tissue somewhere in the body.

It is most unfortunate, in my opinion, that the classification of food known as fat and repugnant term 'fat' are used interchangeably by most people. Although fat yields more calories per gram (9 as compared to 4) than carbohydrates, the body is far more able to utilize the energy from a gram of fat than it is that of a gram of carbohydrate, because the digestion-absorption-conversion cycle of fat is about 15 times longer than that of a sugar (carbohydrate). Because of this time factor, the fat is more efficiently utilized and is not stored as adipose tissue. On the other hand, the carbohydrate food places an immediate demand upon the body to do something, either exercise vigorously so that we can burn this up, or else convert it to fat for future use in time of need.

For years, nutritionists have stated that carbohydrates provide a 'protein sparing' action — in other words, if you don't eat carbohydrates, the body will convert your muscle tissue and other protein tissue into sugar in order to maintain the blood sugar level. This is true — BUT ONLY IF you don't have an ounce of fat or adipose tissue on your frame. What has been overlooked is the fact that the body will first turn to the stored fat, storage fat converts to glucose easier and provides more energy (calories) than does protein. Fat is the true 'storage fuel' of the body. Therefore, the fear of losing valuable gland and muscle tissue because of a lowered intake of carbohydrates is only true when there is no adipose tissue present — and I know very few thin people who concern themselves with their intake of carbohydrates — they normally use all that is necessary for balanced metabolism.

WHY FAT — THIN?

This brings up another question that has bothered over-weight individuals since the beginning of time. Everyone knows someone who eats prodigious amounts of food — of any and every variety — and never gets fat. The overweight person standing behind them in the smorgasbord line puts half as much food on his plate and gains half a pound. What goes here — is it glands? The answer is made up of three distinct possibilities as I see it.

1. Type A — The individual who is able to consume large amounts of food may have a hyperactive glandular system which immediately burns up the energy released from the

food eaten. Or Type A may exercise a great deal, thus demanding more fuel just to maintain status quo.

2. Type B — This individual may consume moderate amounts of food but is consistently fighting a weight problem. The problem may lie in an underactive glandular system, particularly thyroid, which will just not use up the potential energy released from the food — and that excess wil then be stored as fat. Another possibility is just plain lack of exercise — probably more prevalent.

3. Type C — All of us are biochemial individuals. We see drawings of what the heart and kidneys look like; but when an autopsy is performed, only rarely is the size and shape of heart identical to the textbook. This fact can have a strong bearing on the overweight problem. Theoretically, there are 21 feet of small intestine in each of us, through which we absorb nutrients from the food we have eaten. Consider the individual who has 23 feet of intestinal tract for absorption — he has the potential for absorbing 10% more with each meal he eats. Therefore, if he eats an identical amount of food and exercises exactly the same as our mythical normal who only has 21 feet of intestines for absorption, he will gain weight just like compound interest at the bank — in nine years he can double his weight. The individual who has a short intestine of only 19 feet will be capable of eating more because his body is rather inefficient by comparison at extracting nutrients from the food eaten.

PHYSICAL REASONS

In addition to the aforementioned possibilities, there are other reasons for consistent weight gain. One of the most prevalent is constipation. Constipation slows down the tract time which allows the food to be more efficiently absorbed — thus more calories and more possibility that part of that food will be converted to fat. Many overweight individuals have found that my 'Roto Rooter' breakfast (outlined later) can be of immediate benefit in initiating a weight loss that is permanent. Such a breakfast speeds up the 'tract time' and, for the reasons outlined previously, prevents an excessively long period of time for absorption of food. It also has the side benefit of preventing resorption from the large intestine (colon) of the putrefactive bacteria which abound in constipation. This toxic resorption is often the cause of headaches and many minor aches and pains.

An often unexplained phenomenon associated with overweight is the 'craving' for food which can sweep over an individual with such an intensity that it is practically impossible to resist. What causes it? Even more important, what can be done to control it? There are two factors involved:

A. Low Blood Sugar

B. An inadequate supply of essential nutrients such as minerals, vitamins, proteins, etc.

In the low blood sugar situation, a very serious glandular imbalance is present, and a rejuvenation of these glands with restoration to normal function is necessary before the cravings can be overcome. If you feel that this is your problem, I recommend you read my chapter on HYPO-GLYCEMIA for full and complete details. An easy way to determine your tendency toward hypoglycemia (low blood sugar) is to answer the following questions:

1. *Do you wake up depressed, irritable?*
2. *Does stress and strain exhaust you?*
3. *Do you have midmorning and midafternoon letdowns?*
4. *Do you get nervous if a meal is late?*
5. *Does your family consider you an emotional yo-yo? (spirits change very rapidly)*
6. *Sometimes feel you can't think straight?*
7. *Does eating sweets relieve the symptoms?*

If your answer to any one of these was yes, there is a possibility that you have hypoglycemia, and further checking is advisable.

Another reason for the unexplained craving you might have, is the inadequate intake of nutrients to keep the repair and replacement process going in the body. Such a negative balance will result in the body demanding food in ever increasing quantities in an attempt to secure what it needs to maintain the integrity of the tissues. If the food intake should be of such low quality that the nutrients are still not present, the craving will continue — as will the pointer on your weight scale. One of the means of controlling such body messages is to supplement your diet with a broad spectrum, balanced nutritional supplement. This should contain adequate of all the B Complex vitamins, plenty of vitamins C and E, and even more important, lots of all the minerals. On the recommended program of positive weight loss, instructions are given as to an adequate formula and how to use it daily. The need for some vital minerals can be so critical that children eat plaster off walls and dirt off the ground in an attempt to obtain them.

Protein is another of the food classifications which is often deficient in the diet and produces a craving for more food. An inadequate protein intake will often give the sensation of hunger within a half hour after eating! This usually occurs because a diet made up primarily of carbohydrates leaves the stomach very quickly — often within 15 minutes. Proteins and fats remain in the stomach for extended periods of time — often up to 4 or 5 hours, thus the appestat is depressed and you don't feel hungry.

Many find that the use of a protein drink between meals is an excellent means of satisfying the craving for food which so often leads to a snack high in sugar. A variety of such protein powders to make up the protein drink are available in your health food store. *Caution:* Read the labels very carefully to make sure that the product you are considering does not contain sugar in one of its many forms — dextrose, lactose, raw sugar, honey, corn sweeteners, etc. These concentrated forms of sugar cannot benefit you, so avoid them.

FASTING

Not many years ago, you were either a religious fanatic or a health food nut if you considered fasting. Today, doctors use it routinely in any number of disease conditions as a method of restoring the body to normalcy. The overweight individual can use the principles of fasting to a great advantage with an unusual amount of safety. Several physiological changes occur in fasting:

1. Digestive tract has a chance to totally cleanse itself of accumulated waste and putrefactive bacteria.
2. Because the universal solvent, water, is used rather copiously in most fasts, kidney and blood stream purification takes place. This is impossible under ordinary eating patterns and habits.
3. A mental clarity is achieved that is not possible under the constant bombardment of chemicals and food additives.
4. The stomach has a chance to shrink back to a normal size, thus making it easier to control the quantity you eat.
5. Eating habits are broken, so that when you come off the fast, it is easy to begin anew with good habits of eating.

I highly recommend the Liver-Kidney-Bowel Cleansing Fast explained later in this book as an extremely efficient means of preparing the body for new health patterns. A new broom is supposed to sweep clean — the fast will cleanse your body without weakening it and at the same time start you on your way to a slimmer figure with an average weight loss of from 5 to 7 pounds the first three days! Such a beginning is very encouraging to anyone on a weight reducing program and keeps the spirits up, so more success can be achieved — and success in this case means health, the greatest wealth of all.

EXERCISE

No program would be complete without a discussion on the effect exercise has on weight loss. First of all, let us understand that I feel it is absolutely necessary that one have an exercise routine — not only to lose weight but also to maintain good health. In this day of convenience everything, only the athlete and the physical laborer sustain good tissue tone by their normal daily activities. The rest of us exercise our brain cells, and often are so lethargic by the time we get home in the evening, the obvious thing to do is flop in an easy chair in front of the TV and enjoy our exercise in a vicarious fashion. And woe to us, the result has been an astounding 4 out of every 10 Americans is overweight!

WHEN AND HOW TO EXERCISE

One factor that I do not believe is emphasized enough, is the importance of timing in exercise — particularly when you are trying to control your appetite and also your weight. The best time to exercise for this purpose is *just before eating*. Let me explain the physiology behind that statement.

We earlier discussed the fact that the body converts part

96

of the excess fuel derived from the food we eat to a substance called glycogen, which is subsequently stored in the liver and muscle tissue for immediate conversion back to glucose in time of need. Exercise is a time of need, therefore the conversion takes place then and the blood sugar level is elevated to supply the fuel. When I refer to exercise at this time, I am not talking about a 60-minute tennis match or 50 laps in the pool. I am talking about a controlled physical exertion of from 5 to 10 minutes, no more than 10 minutes before a meal. If you eat at 8 AM, begin your exercise at 7:40 AM. The resultant rise in blood sugar will decrease your appetite, permitting you closer adherance to a proper eating program.

The biggest question pertains to the proper exercise for such a short period of time. Some prefer calisthenics, others isometrics, push and pull equipment is the in thing now, but I have found the most effective complete body exercise for these short periods of time to be a miniature trampoline. Several models are out and I suggest you investigate the possibility of such a unit. It is readily stored in your home, you need not disrobe to use it, and the medical reports on the effect are extremely salutatory. Remember to use it before each meal, if at all possible, and for certain before the traditional large dinner. A side benefit is the alertness and desire to meet daily tasks when you do this regularly before breakfast.

POSITIVE MENTAL ATTITUDE

It is my opinion that the age of psychologist and the psychiatrist is ebbing away. We are becoming more aware of the 'power within' each and every one of us. A few preparatory steps taken to marshall that power you have, will make your weight loss program so much easier to follow. Success will be assured, and that is what you are after — a successful, non-recurring weight loss which will restore your confidence and add untold years of productive happy years to your life.

The method found successful by many is to type out the following statements on a card:

I WILL

1. I have determined that my proper weight is ___ lbs.
2. To attain this I will do the following:
   a. Cleanse my body by fasting as needed.
   b. Exercise for a least 5 minutes before each meal.
   c. Follow the food selection chart as outlined.
   d. Use food supplements to alleviate hidden hunger.
   e. Practice my mental recharging each morning and night.
3. In gratitude for all my blessings, I will conduct myself in such a fashion as to reflect goodness, confidence and consideration for all my fellow mankind.

To achieve mental recharging by the use of this card, the following procedure is recommended:
1. Just before breakfast each morning, sit down in a comfortable chair and spend one minute relaxing your body. This can easily be done by just concentrating on a complete slackening of the muscles of your legs, pelvis, abdomen, arms, shoulders, and neck in that order.
2. Pick up the card and read each statement carefully.
3. Meditate upon the statements on the card, visualize them if you can for a period of one minute.
4. Repeat the above just before dinner.

Sound too simple to be true? Just try that amazing force within your mind for results that will astound you!

The message on the card is a synopsis of what must be done. By now you should know why you are overweight and how to cope with the situation — the only factor remaining is your cooperation. The following pages will give you pertinent information on all of the steps outlined. Put them to use and see how much brighter the sun shines through!

FOOD SUPPLEMENTS

My opinion on these substances has remained firm over the years. I feel they are an absolute necessity and I am strongly opposed to 'fragmented nutrition' where the product used is not a complete vitamin and mineral complex. The following ingredients are a must in my book when you are choosing a supplement:

Vitamin A	25,000IU	Inositol	60mg
Vitamin D	400IU	Folic Acid	400mcg
Vitamin E	400IU	Biotin	100mcg
Vitamin C	1,200mg	Calcium	1000mg
Vitamin B-1	60mg	Magnesium	400mg
Vitamin B-2	60mg	Phosphorus	150mg
Vitamin B-6	60mg	Potassium	99mg
Vitamin B-12	100mcg	Iron	15mg
Niacin	30mg	Iodine	225 mcg
Niacinamide	30mg	Copper	2mg
Pantothenic Acid	100mg	Chromium	500mcg
PABA	60mg	Manganese	15mg
Choline	60 mg	Zinc	15mg
		Selenium	100mcg

These are minimum quantities for a daily intake and some formulae may have added digestants, herbs and other food factors which enhance the product. Formula such as the above are available from your health food store vitamin supplier, so read your label and get the best.

RESTORE GLAND FUNCTION

The use of an all-inclusive vitamin and mineral preparation will assist greatly to normalize glandular function. It has been mentioned previously that in some instances stress and other factors have so depleted the glandular functions that sluggishness of these glands contributes to the overweight problem. Because of an intensive study, we now know that certain factors within each cell control its function, and perhaps even more important, its rebuilding process. They are called the DNA and RNA factors.

When a gland is sluggish, it is usually because new cells are not replacing the old ones as they die off. Two factors within the cell, DNA and RNA, work together in this all important restructuring of cells. When DNA and RNA are behind in their regenerative work, the deterioration of an organ, gland or system in the body begins. Such deterioration has profound effect on the body as a whole, it can affect the mind, the physical capacity can be greatly reduced, and very importantly, our ability to convert fat to glycogen to sugar for energy is reduced. This can raise havoc with a weight control program.

Researchers have found that DNA-RNA factors can be transferred from one animal to another; at least the present evidence has led scientists to postulate that if you eat pancreas substance, your pancreas will renew its cells at a faster rate, thus being capable of performing its functions more efficiently. It has been my experience that the use of a multi-glandular concentrate tablet can be of inestimable value. Such a product can be obtained without prescription from your local health food store.

FEMALE

Ovarian Substance	60mg
Whole Pituitary Substance	20mg
Adrenal Substance	60mg
Thymus Substance	60mg
Pancreas Substance	60mg
Kidney Substance	60mg
Heart Substance	60mg
Ribonucleic Acid (RNA)	60mg

MALE

Prostate Substance	60mg
Whole Pituitary Substance	20mg
Adrenal Substance	60mg
Thymus Substance	60mg
Pancreas Substance	60mg
Kidney Substance	60mg
Heart Substance	60mg
Ribonucleic Acid (RNA)	60mg

PROTEIN DRINK

The diet suggested with this program calls for the use of a protein drink between meals and at bedtime, if necessary to control hunger and snacking. Caution was necessary to avoid the use of protein products which contained sugars. What kind of protein product should one consider?

First of all, remember that a protein is not judged by its total protein content, but by its efficiency ratio. Thus a protein containing only 70% total protein may benefit the body more than one which has a 96% protein content. This efficiency ratio is determined by the balance of essential amino acids in the product. If one is quite low, then the efficiency is lowered because in order for protein to be utilized properly in the body, all essential amino acids must be present at the same time.

For this basic reason, a protein made up of multiple sources is usually considered superior to a single source protein. Also, animal source proteins, such as glandular material, casein, eggs, etc. are considered more efficient than vegetable proteins. It must be noted that many consider a blend of animal and vegetable sources the ideal product. You will find this combination type product where you buy your food supplemets.

For proper digestion, we recommend that the protein drink be made with a vegetable juice or raw milk, and not fruit juices, as this protein — carbohydrate combination can lead to indigestion. Most of these powders mix readily by stirring with a spoon, shaking in a closed container or using your blender.

SUGGESTED DIET

Branola Breakfast: (Sometimes called "ROTO-ROOTER BREAKFAST")
½cup raw millers bran
½cup granola (no sugar added)
4 tablespoons cream (raw preferred)
2 tablespoons full fat yogurt (unflavored)
Add water to desired consistency. This combination of ingredients does several things for you:

1. They furnish you with high fiber which speeds up the digestive tract time, therefore less efficient absorption of calories, less tendency toward constipation, less toxins.

2. By being high in fats, they give you a longer sensation of fullness and offer a source of energy that is used more completely by the body than carbohydrates, which are often stored as fats.

3. The yogurt helps to sweeten up and restore the friendly bacteria in the lower tract.

Mid-Morning and Mid-Afternoon Snack — this is to be

used if you have letdown at these times or have a craving for food. Mix together:

  2 rounded tablespoons protein powder
  6 - 8 oz. raw milk or vegetable juice

Lunch: Meat, fish, eggs, or cheese; vegetables as indicated on chart, nuts or seeds.

Dinner: Soup if desired (not thickened with flour), vegetables and meat as allowed, one slice of whole grain bread and butter.

Beverages: Most desirable is water, herb teas and cereal coffee are fine. No sugar, please.

SELECTION CHART

Choice Group:

Meat .... Veal, beef, lamb, fish, poultry are the best choices. Ham, bacon, sausage and other processed meats should be eliminated.

Fruits .... Apricots, apples, berries, melons, peaches, pears, pineapple, tangerines, grapefruit, oranges, cantaloupe, strawberries, watermelon, plums.

Juices .... Any unsweetened fruit or vegetable juice, except grape or prune juice. Best fresh.

Vegetables ..... Any vegetable except those listed below.

Beverages ...... Herb tea, cereal coffee substitute. No sugar added.

Desserts .... Fruits — preferably eaten 3 hours after meal.

Note: Fruits should be raw or cooked without sugar. If you use canned, be sure they are packed in water. Best raw.

Avoid Group:

Alcoholic and

Soft Drinks .... Wines, cordials, cocktails, beer, whiskey, cola drinks, pop of all kinds, ginger ale, club soda.

Vegetables ..... Hominy, rice, yams, potato (except raw or baked twice weekly), corn, dried beans.

Juices .... Grape juice and prune juice.

Prepared Foods .. White flour, bakery products, spaghetti, macaroni, noodles, gravies.

Beverages ...... Coffee and tea.

Desserts .... Candy and other sugar sweets, such as cake, pie, pastries, custard, jello, ice cream, sherbets, puddings.

CLASSIFICATION OF FOODS
According to Carbohydrate Content)
VEGETABLES

3 PERCENT	6 PERCENT	15 PERCENT	20 PERCENT	25 PERCENT
Asparagus	Beans, string	Artichokes	Beans, dried	Rice, boiled
Bean sprouts	Beets	Beans, Kidney	Beans, Lima	Potato, sweet
Beet greens	Brussel sprouts	Hominy	Corn	Yams
Broccoli	Carrots	Oyster plant	Potato, white	
Cabbage	Chives	Parsnips		
Cauliflower	Collards	Peas, green		
Celery	Dandelion			
Chard, Swiss	greens			
Cucumber	Eggplant			
Endive	Kale			
Lettuce	Kohlrabi			
Mushrooms	Leeks			
Mustard	Okra			
greens	Onions			
Radishes	Parsley			
Sauerkraut	Peppers, red			
Spinach	Pimento			
Squash	Pumpkin			
Tomatoes	Rutabagas			
Tomato juice	Turnips			
Turnip greens				
Water cress				

104

FRUITS

3 PERCENT	6 PERCENT	15 PERCENT	20 PERCENT	25 PERCENT
Cantaloupe	Apricots	Apples	Bananas	
Rhubarb	Blackberries	Blueberries	Figs	
Strawberries	Cranberries	Cherries	Prunes	
Watermelon	Currants	Grapes		
	Gooseberries	Kumquats		
	Grapefruit	Loganberries		
	Guava	Mangoes		
	Melons	Mulberries		
	Lemons	Pears		
	Limes	Pineapple		
	Oranges	Pomegranates		
	Papayas			
	Peaches			
	Plums			
	Raspberries			
	Tangerines			

In making your choice of vegetables, you may use all the 3% and 6% selections you wish every day. Twice weekly choose one from the 15% or 25% groups as a change.

In making your choice of fruits, it is desirable that you limit the amount to one 3% selection during the first days of your diet. As you progress, other choices can be made.

Chapter 7

ALLERGIES

Allergies, like many other health problems or abnormalities, can be caused by mental and emotional disturbances or stress. These are by no means the only cause, but we should understand this aspect in order that we can see the tie between our emotional and our chemical balance.

First of all, in all emotional stress situations, the sympathetic nervous system is called upon to respond to the stimulus, whatever it may be. The sympathetic nervous system has sometimes been called the sympatho-adrenal system because of the importance the adrenal glands play in the function.

It is an amazing chain reaction that occurs when a stimulation such as fear, anger, change in temperature, or even an overactive imagination is received by the nervous system. Heart action is speeded up, blood pressure is raised by a constricting action on the blood vessels, breathing becomes more rapid, and digestive functions slow down almost to a stop. Most of these changes are due to hormones released from the adrenals, which begin their action within split seconds after stimulation.

These same reactions often occur when certain drugs or toxins are introduced into the body. This type of body function changes are 'defense mechanisms.' They make us ready to accommodate the needs we have under various conditions.

Now just imagine the body that does not respond as I have described because the adrenals do not pour out the hormones necessary to create the changes. A good example can be described — a cat had his adrenal nerve supply removed. The following changes were noted:

1. Capacity for muscular activity decreased by 35%.
2. Animal did not defend itself against cold by erection of hair and vasoconstriction of cutaneous blood vessels.
3. Animal had to be kept in a warm room or body temperature fell.
4. Animal went into shock when exposed to emotional excitement. (This is important as it shows the necessity of our response to the stress of life. If we don't respond by raising our blood pressure, our blood sugar, and our oxygen supply, then we have not accommodated the needs that the stimulus placed on our body and serious consequences result.)
5. Animal developed allergic reactions to many foods and other chemicals that previously were not considered allergens.

Such changes represent no adrenal function and are severe, but decreased function would logically represent similar type symptom patterns — including decreased energy, allergies, temperature adaptation problems, etc. Since we are primarily concerned with allergies and the foreign substances which enter the blood stream and are not handled properly which produce the allergy, let us trace the beginning of an allergy.

A foreign protein — it can be pollen, drugs, foods, chemicals, etc. — enters the blood stream in an undenatured state. The offending substance may enter in any of a number of ways — by the alimentary tract, through the lungs, through the skin or a break in the skin, or by injection. Immediately signals are sent out for antibodies to attack this foreign organism and destroy it. The signals produce a number of hormones which facilitate the antibody release. Most of these hormones originate in the adrenal glands.

When the antibodies attack the foreign protein, the first purpose is to denature it by chemical action. This chemical action produces a by-product known as histamine. Histamine is a tissue toxin in that it causes vaso-dilation (the characteristic blood vessel enlargement which causes flushing sensations and a redness of the skin), and increased permeability of the blood vessel wall, allowing fluids to escape and thus bringing about localized edema or swelling. In allergies, this can exhibit itself as congestion in the respiratory tract or raised wheals on the skin, or an itching anywhere on the body. More serious internal effects can occur, including mental derangements, headaches, gastrointestinal upsets, diarrhea, asthma, sinusitis, etc.

Food allergies can often be corrected by increasing the amount of digestive enzymes which break down the raw protein into amino acids. This can be done by the use of supplemental enzymes available from your health food store.

Drug and cosmetic allergies can usually be controlled by eliminating the use of the offending substance. We should be aware that many substances are absorbed through the skin directly into the blood stream. The tremendous amount of chemicals used in cosmetics are the cause of many problems in the area of the face — headaches from chemical dyes, sinusitis, sore throat type symptoms from perfumes or facial cremes, and the immediate redness and inflammation experienced when a cosmetic containing a chemical you react to is applied.

HYPERKINESIS or HYPERACTIVITY

Following the extensive research of Dr. Ben Feingold

(Why Your Child Is Hyperactive), it has now been documented that the cause of the hyper-activity is an allergy — usually to the additives in the foods such as artificial coloring or artificial flavoring. Since children respond so rapidly to any proper treatment, Dr. Feingold (and now many others) was able to show a dramatic improvement in children who were previously uncontrollable without powerful drugs and had learning problems. The average length of time was less than 10 days after artificial coloring and additives were removed from the diet, and symptoms immediately recurred when just one of the offending products was reintroduced to the diet.

Millions of parents and most certainly the children affected, owe Dr. Feingold a debt that can only be repaid with thankful prayer. No amount of money can repay for the rehabilitation of every one of these children. It is sad to see that his program was not adopted as standard practice by all physicians. All too many are still prescribing the amphetamine drugs which literally turn the children into 'zombies' who are unable to learn properly or adjust properly to their environment. One wonders how many sociopathic criminals were really allergic victims who were unable to understand society or social order.

THE BIG QUESTION

The big question which arises is why are some children allergic to the additives and others are not? Why are some women allergic to cosmetics and others not? Why can some eat strawberries and others not?

I HAVE TO GO BACK TO THE BASIC PREMISE THAT A HEALTHY BODY IS CAPABLE OF NEUTRALIZING THESE TOXIC SUBSTANCES AND A BODY WHICH HAS MALFUNCTIONING DEFENSE MECHANISMS CANNOT. THE EMPHASIS IN ALLERGIES MUST

BE ON BUILDING A HEALTHY BODY, NOT ON TRYING TO USE EVASIVE TACTICS BY ELIMINATING ALL THE ALLERGENS. It only makes common sense that such allergens as chemicals, drugs, cosmetics, etc., be elimintated, but if the body is not strengthened, the individual will become allergic to other entities.

One of the most frustrating experiences an allergy victim has is the skin patch test. Here various substances are taped or applied to the skin and if you react by redness of the area, then you are allergic to that particular substance. Treatment then consists of desensitizing you to the specific allergen or allergens. After a 12 to 24 month course of weekly injections, you find that the old allergies are no more, but now the patch test reveals a whole new set which must go through the same procedure. It seems like you never get well, just change allergies!

While we are on the subject, most allergy victims are not very resistant to other disorders either. They often 'catch' everything that comes along, are anemic, and have low energy levels. All of these symptoms tie into that discussion we just had on the adrenal glands. When your adrenals are not working well, you lose stamina rapidly.

ANTI-HISTAMINE

Everyone with an allergy and most others are familiar with the term anti-histamine. This substance acts to neutralize the existing histamine and presto! the symptoms are relieved. Many associate anti-histamine with tablets, capsules, and sprays which are purchased in the drug store.

We should never forget how wondrous the human mechanism really is. Since histamine is a natural by product of the denaturing process of a foreign protein in the body, natural anti-histamine is produced by the liver under normal circumstances. If the liver is 'plugged up' with fatty tissue and an excess of toxins which it cannot neutralize, therefore storing them within itself rather than allowing them out in the general circulation, there is a possibility of inadequate secretion of anti-histamine and allergies result.

In such cases, allergies clear up miraculously when the liver is detoxified. I have outlined a Liver-Kidney-Bowel detoxifying fast later in this book and heartily recommend it for all who suffer from allergies.

BACK TO THE ADRENALS

Almost all allergies have been treated with temporary success by the use of the adrenal hormones ACTH and cortisone. Now if the adrenals were not involved in allergies, such treatment would not be successful, so let's accept the fact that the adrenals are malfunctioning. Why are they not functioning properly? The answer usually lies in one area in my opinion — poor nutrition.

Studies have indicated that people suffering from allergies are woefully deficient in many nutritional factors, and when these nutritional factors are supplied, the allergies disappear. For example, children suffering from asthma, hives, or eczema markedly improved when the only change in their diet was the addition of B Complex factors.

Another study had a 100% recovery rate from bronchial asthma and allergic eczema in 32 children who were put on a high protein, moderate fat, very low carbohydrate program supplemented with a broad spectrum vitamin-mineral supplement.

I have personally observed many recoveries from allergies and have noted that the younger the sufferer the quicker they recover. It seems that as you allow the deterioration of the adrenals to progress, it takes longer to rejuvenate and regenerate them. Instead of taking two months for a recovery as the children in the previously reported study, it might be four or six months recovery period. But, as an allergy victim will attest, it was worth it all!

PANTOTHENIC ACID

A very important adrenal hormone, cortisone, cannot be produced without an adequate supply of pantothenic acid in the system. We know that cortisone is essential in preventing the symptoms of allergies. In fact, if an allergen is injected into an allergic person, the subsequent allergies are relieved by injections of cortisone. But if the diet of the allergic victim is supplemented with pantothenic acid for a period of time, the allergic reaction also disappears. Amounts of as little as 250 mg. per day have been effective but the best results were obtained by the use of up to 3,000 mg. daily.

SYMPTOMS OF DEFICIENCY

Symptoms of pantothenic acid deficiency include a host of seemingly unrelated malfunctions but they are all connected to the sympatho-adrenal nervous system which relies so much on the adrenal glands. Here is a partial list of symptoms:

Fatigue
Listlessness
Poor Appetite
Digestive Disturbances
Headaches
Recurrent Respiratory Infections

Irritability
Nervousness
Mental Depression
Quarrelsomeness
Increased Need for Sleep

Because of our peculiar biochemical individuality, the needs for certain nutrients may vary by as much as 3,000 per cent. What this means is that some may function very well on 100 mg. daily of pantothenic acid while others would need 3,000 mg. to attain the same level of well-being.

VITAMIN B-6

Reports of anti-histamine effects from vitamin B-6 are another demonstration of the biochemical individuality thesis. We have no 'magic bullet' that answers all our needs in a particular problem. Since magnesium 'spares' B-6 in the body, a deficiency of this mineral can also be a factor. Under most circumstances the amount of B-6 used is from 25 to 100 mg. daily.

VITAMIN C

Another vitamin with anti-histamine properties, vitamin C has been used in dosages of 2,000 mg. daily in the treatment of such allergies as asthma, pollen induced allergies, and allergic coryza (runny, stuffed nose). It is very interesting to note that in animals able to manufacture their own vitamin C, an equivalent amount for humans would be a requirement of from 3,000 to 5,000 mg. daily. Many of the tests of vitamin C and its effect on malfunctions of the body have used dosages far too small to be considered effective.

Another benefit that vitamin C furnishes is its protection against cell membrane permeability. Increased cell wall permeability is a factor in allergies because the foreign proteins have easier access to the cell under such conditions. While we are on the subject of cell permeability, vitamin E plays a role in this, so an intake of at least 400 IU daily is suggested. And vitamin A should not be left out because it protects and strengthens the skin and the mucous membranes lining the respiratory and genito-urinary tract.

HYPOGLYCEMIA and ALLERGIES

Very often diagnosed allergies are almost instantaneously relieved by the use of a hypoglycemic diet with adrenal support. In fact, a whole book entitled "Goodbye Allergies" was written on the subject. For further information on the subject please see the section entitled 'Hypoglycemia'. I have often stressed the fact that the 'Carbohydrate Intolerant Diet' used by the hypoglycemic is an ideal diet for many of the ills of mankind and could only benefit someone who chose to follow it.

The very close relationship between allergies and hypoglycemia is due to the common tie of malfunctioning adrenals. In both cases, when this failing is corrected, the symptoms disappear and all seems to be well. The important part, of course, is to be sure that biochemical balance is maintained in the body. Then the stage is never set up for disease entities like allergies and hypoglycemia to step in.

PROGRAM

If you have an allergy and desire to allow your body to heal itself with a little intelligent help, you might consider the following:

1. Help your adrenals to function properly by offering them a smorgasbord of nutritional factors. I have outlined a suggested formula at the end of this chapter

which would contain such concentrates in the amounts I feel adequate.

2. To further stimulate the adrenals, provide them with adrenal DNA, commonly referred to as adrenal nucleoprotein.

3. If it is a food related allergy, add a digestive enzyme supplement to each meal. It is often best to use several tablets of such an enzyme with each meal for about one week, then gradually reduce the intake by one tablet each meal. This procedure will soon show you if enzymes are really helping because as you reduce the intake you will eventually reach the point where symptoms return and you know the enzyme level is too low.

4. Common sense will tell you that adequate rest and freedom from excessive emotional strain will assist your recovery. When present, your need for certain nutrients takes a real upswing.

5. If your body is not releasing adequate anti-histamine from the liver, you should go on a Liver-Kidney-Bowel Cleansing Fast. This is outlined later in detail.

6. After cleansing your liver, the ideal way to choose your food is to follow the Creative Restoration Diet, also outlined later.

SUGGESTED ENZYME FORMULA

Betaine Hydrochloride ..	120mg	Pepsin	65mg
Pancreatin	150mg	Lipase	100mg
Bile Extract	120mg	Papain	100mg

SUGGESTED SUPPLEMENT FORMULA

Pantothenic Acid	2,000mg	Inositol	60mg
Vitamin C	2,200mg	Folic Acid	400mcg

Adrenal Nucleoprotein	390mg	Biotin	100mcg
Vitamin A	10,000IU	Calcium	1000mg
Vitamin D	400IU	Magnesium	400mg
Vitamin E	400IU	Phosphorus	150mg
Vitamin B-1	60mg	Potassium	99mg
Vitamin B-2	60mg	Iron	15mg
Vitamin B-6	60mg	Iodine	225mcg
Vitamin B-12	100mcg	Copper	2mg
Niacin	30mg	Chromium	500mcg
Niacinamide	30mg	Manganese	15mg
PABA	60mg	Zinc	15mg
Choline	60mg		

These are minimum quantities for a daily intake and some formulae may have added digestants, herbs and other food factors which enhance the product. Formula such as the above are available from your health food store or vitamin supplier, so read your label and get the best.

Chapter 8

ACNE

For the average acne sufferer, "the wonders of modern medicine" is a particularly hollow phrase. The only "wonder" is why so little has been done to combat a condition that attacks 80 percent of the teenage population and hundreds of thousands of adults.

Acne is a particularly vicious condition, with physical disfigurement and emotionally crippling consequences. Because of the evident blemishes, many are ashamed and even become anti-social because of a condition which I feel can be, at worst, controlled, and at best cleared up never to return with just a little care on the part of the victim. Although common opinion would have you believe that acne is only for the teenager, many adults even up to the 60s have mild to serious acne problems.

Many observers have told of the beautiful complexions of the Latin races, other comments have been, "Italians just don't get pimples." Surveys done by the National Institutes of Health and others have indicated that Okinawa, Japan, Formosa, and Korea show less than five percent incidence of acne. On the other hand, the Alaskan Indian in the interior has ten times as much acne as the Eskimo on the coast.

DIET IS THE KEY

A rather exciting fact comes to the fore when you move any of the low acne incidence individuals to the United

States and feed him the American diet. The descendants immediately have acne at the same rate as other American teenagers.

Diet is the only common denominator that explains why acne varies so widely. It is not race, it is not climate, it is not external cleanliness, but it is the *kind* of food one consumes.

Now comes the problem — if we search the literature and stop eating everything that is suspected of causing acne, you not only would have a very limited diet, but might be left with only water — distilled at that. Let's try to cut through the inconsistencies and find a rational diet that will first of all help prevent acne, and secondly help clear up existing cases.

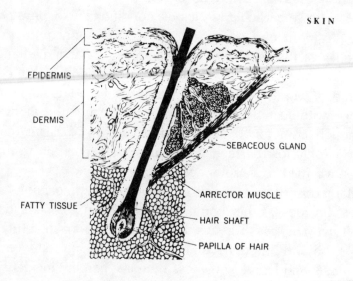

SKIN

HOW DOES ACNE START?

In most individuals, acne begins right around the onset of puberty. In the schematic drawing above, we see a cross section of the skin. Please note the sebaceous glands which are in the dermis, or second layer of skin, containing blood vessels, nerves, hair roots and the sebaceous glands.

Although there is much controversy regarding acne, everyone seems to agree on one point — that an excess secretion of the sebaceous gland is associated with acne. This gland secretes a thin oil which migrates to the surface of the skin to keep it smooth, pliable, and young looking. A hormone called testosterone, which is mainly present in the male but is also present in the female, stimulates the secretion of more oil than usual from the sebaceous gland during puberty. This extra oil has a tendency to accumulate in the skin follicles (tiny, sac-like recesses in the skin) at which time bacteria, which are always present, begin to feed off the oil. The digestion of the oil causes it to break down into fatty acids which may cause the cells that line the follicle to stick together. As a result, the opening of the follicles, called pores can become plugged or impacted with dead cells. Now the bacteria have an ideal arena for further growth, creating more waste cells and further impactions. This is soon evident as the whitehead, blackhead, cyst or pustule so characteristic of acne.

WHY TETRACYCLINE IS SO POPULAR

The use of the antibiotic tetracycline is a very popular treatment for acne because it tends to destroy the bacteria in the whitehead, blackhead, or pustule. The obvious fallacy in this approach is very evident upon stopping the treatment. In almost every instance the pimples start up again and eventually the antibiotic becomes ineffective after repeated use because the bacteria builds up a tolerance to it.

So where does that leave us? If testosterone causes excess secretion, should we try to diminish the hormone? That approach is not practical since the male sex hormone is absolutely essential for the development of the male characteristics. Now, as we mentioned before, testosterone

119

is also present in small amounts in the female, those girls who have slightly elevated levels will be more prone to acne than those who have lower levels. (It should be noted that a certain amount of estrogen, the female hormone, is also present in all males.) This also explains why more acne is present in males than in females on an overall level.

Another concept holds that if you cleanse your skin with a bacteriocidal cleanser on a twice daily basis, the bacteria will not have a chance to work on the oil in the skin follicle and start the whole vicious cycle. This is partly effective in certain cases, but there is quite some concern that this constant application of external germicides can and does result in absorption through the skin of chemicals which may have detrimental effects on the body as a whole. So, I agree we have to have something to control the bacteria if acne exists, but the problem of a safe germicide which is not resorbed into the system as a foreign chemical to disrupt other systems, must be overcome before I am satisfied.

ACNE AND STRESS

There is a popular theory that the stress of teenage life is at least partly responsible for acne. There is no question that the early teen years are exceptionally stressful, but then, as many of us have painfully learned, no more stressful than those adult years which follow. I do not discount some validity in stress as a factor — but just want to make it clear that I do not feel it is a primary or sole cause of acne.

Stress does affect the whole human mechanism, and thus can affect acne. When the human mechanism is subjected to excess stress, the adrenal glands are stimulated to increase their production of androgen hormone which is similar to testosterone in its stimulation of oil production by the sebaceous glands. Since there is an individual tolerance factor, the mere presence of stress does not automatically produce acne. Those individuals who have adequate reservoirs of the B Complex vitamins often accommodate tremendous loads of stress without triggering unusual adrenal response. It is my opinion that this factor alone is well worth considering by all who are involved in the world today which has to be considered a time of high stress. Your attention to the use of a B Complex could mean the difference between "coping" or succumbing to the erratic behavior and possible skin problems other than acne — such as 'shingles' so often associated with high stress today.

Another negative reaction which affects the skin during stress is the fact that in the individual who does not adjust to stress, because of poor nutrition or whatever reason, the blood supply to the surface of the skin is very measurably diminished. Without a good blood supply the natural healing processes of the body are seriously hindered allowing further infection. A good example of this is the blanched appearance of a person who is angry, or who has just received bad news, or has been frightened. The pale appearance is from the loss of blood supply to the outer layers of the skin as the tiny capillaries are constricted.

I would like to emphasize again the need to pay attention to proper nutrition, particularly those nutrients which affect the adrenal glands — pantothenic acid, vitamin C, and potassium.

VITAMIN A

An external treatment using vitamin A acid and benzyl peroxide is at present the most popular medical means of controlling acne. The dermatologists using this approach stress that their treatment is not a cure, but only a control. The rationale behind the treatment is as follows:

1. The vitamin A acid acts on the cells of the follicle in such a way as to prevent their sticking together, thus inhibiting the formation of an impaction which produces the "pimple."

2. Benzyl peroxide seems to be an extremely effective agent for the destruction of the acne bacteria. This is applied in the evening while the vitamin A acid is applied in the morning. Although this treatment is very effective on a more or less immediate basis (4 to 8 weeks) it must be continued or the acne condition returns. It is still a mystery to me why specialization in the healing arts is so highly revered in our society today. I do not wish to detract from the high quality of knowledge that specialists attain, but I often feel they don't "see the forest for the trees." The program which I used successfully for some years and have helped other physicians to put into their practice runs an interesting parallel to the work with vitamin A acid and benzyl peroxide therapy. It is, however, my opinion that the approach I used is more physiologic in concept in that it considers acne as a systemic disease, not just one of the skin, and with proper application can have far more long term effects because it tends to eliminate the cause instead of topically eliminating the symptoms temporarily.

ACNE CONTROL PROGRAM

Many years ago, when the first real serious acne patient was brought to me, I was deeply impressed with the seriousness of the situation. A young man, 14 years of age, his face so covered with cysts and pustules that he refused to look at anyone when he was in their presence, his back and chest a weeping mass of large open pustules that did not allow him to wear anything but a T-shirt, stood before me. I was shocked, but tried desperately not to show it. The mother told me he refused to go to school and always went to his room when any visitors came to the house. You can imagine the psychological effects on this young man!

I knew I had to help his body cleanse itself of some of those toxins, so I started with what is now known as my Liver-Kidney-Bowel Cleansing Fast. Since this program automatically eliminates all "junk food," I also accomplished that goal without any difficulty. At the end of the third day we began introducing foods slowly — per the instructions in the diet which are reprinted at the end of this book. I also added 150,000 IU of vitamin A from fish liver oil on a daily basis and he was instructed to begin taking a broad spectrum multi-vitamin and mineral supplement that satisfied my requirements for potency and balance.

Externally we suggested he use an adsorbent clay which picks up (like a sponge) dead protein matter from the skin when left on for a few minutes. Then he used a zinc ointment as a germicide and astringent topically. Once a day vitamin E ointment was applied to all the areas to speed up healing.

Within six weeks a new person came into my office. The change was so dramatic that I did not even recognize him as the same young man who had first walked in. There was still some evidence of a skin problem, but so slight as to be inconsequential. His chest and back had almost completely cleared with just signs of healing remaining. This single case brought young people from as far away as Canada to my office for help with acne type problems. Shortly after we began this approach, Dr. Frank's work on external application of RNA in the form of a cream was published. The message was very clear to me that RNA would assist in bringing normal skin appearance to the areas of scars and pits of the acne victim. So I began using a combination of RNA and vitamin E as the night-time application and the results were even better on the lesions left after the inflammation had been cleared up. By combining the two we saved one application and saved some money for the patient also.

QUESTIONS MOST COMMONLY ASKED BY PHYSICIANS AND ACNE VICTIMS REGARDING THIS PROGRAM.

Q. Why do you use such high amounts of vitamin A and are you not concerned that this amount may be toxic?

A. You will recall the rationale of the external vitamin A therapy — the vitamin A helps prevent the sticking together of the lining cells of the skin follicle — which sticking can produce the impaction of the pore, producing acne. By using the vitamin A systemically or internally, we produce the same result as the external application, but for longer lasting periods of time. Vitamin A is a fat soluble vitamin and can be stored in the body. Once we have supplied the need to prevent the acne, the body can begin storing it for future use. As to its possible toxicity, I can honestly say that I have never seen a case of natural vitamin A toxicity, nor do I know any physicians who have. The cases cited by some of the 'scare mongers' of vitamin A causing all kinds of problems are all cases of exceptionally high amounts of vitamin A (500,000 to 3,000,000 IU per day) and always of the synthetic variety. Even these records show that the discontinuance of the high dosages of the synthetic variety of vitamin A produced complete remission of all symptoms within three to ten days. On the other hand, I have a report from the United States Department of Agriculture that says 33% of our teenagers are deficient in vitamin A. A footnote

124

to that statement makes it clear that the 5,000 IU which was used for purposes of testing may well be too low a figure for good health and thus the deficiency of vitamin A among our teenagers may be even greater than one out of three.

Another interesting facet of vitamin A usage by these teenagers was a great increase in fingernail flexibility and growth. I have used this knowledge effectively where individuals were complaining of dry brittle nails. It might also be of some interest to know that I have consumed an average of 250,000 IU of fish liver oil vitamin A every day for the last 15 years. It is the only supplement that assists me in controlling a chronic sinus probem.

Q. Are there any foods which are particularly detrimental to the success of the program?

A. Very definitely! All high sugar containing foods must be eliminated; this includes all soft drinks, pies, cakes, pastries, ice cream, cookies, candy, etc. Refined white flour products should also be eliminated, with emphasis on consuming whole grains, raw vegetables and fruits, eggs, cheese, various meats but refraining from processed meats. These rules and regulations are thoroughly covered in my Creative Restoration Diet.

Q. Can the individual eat nuts and nut butters on your program?

A. They certainly can. We suggest raw nuts and seeds if possible.

Q. Will this program work for the adult acne sufferer as well?

A. Yes it will, but I would rather have a teenager as a patient because they tend to follow instructions better. The basic physiology is the same, so the results are the same.

Q. What is the percentage of results with this program?

A. I can honestly say that I have never seen a case of acne that was not helped to some degree. It has been my experience that if the individual follows the program very closely, he will be very satisfied with the results.

Q. Why do the high sugar foods affect the skin — particularly when it comes to acne?

A. First of all, they are usually foodless foods; they do not contain essential nutrients that the body needs in its daily ecology. Therefore the consumption of these foods substitutes for vitamin, mineral, and protein containing foods which are necessary for the body. They also disrupt the glandular system in the body in that man is not designed to handle heavy concentrations of sugar. When such concentrated sugar containing foods are consumed, erratic blood sugar patterns often result. Such deviations can create glandular crises which may stimulate the androgenic hormones which stimulate extra oil from the sebaceous gland.

Q. How long should one stay on your program?

A. The dietary portion of it should become a way of life. The use of the cleansing and germicidal preparation is something which will also enhance normal skin, so can be used periodically just for maintenance. The RNA and vitamin E creme is also a product which will help to maintain a youthful appearance, so there is no contraindication there — in fact, I have many written testimonials as to the skin softening and rejuvenating effects of this cream.

Q. Can the scars of acne really be removed with this program?

A. Some of the deep, pitted areas will not fully restore to normal, but the skin will become much more soft and pliable so that they will not be nearly as visible. The other areas will be so restored that you will not even know that you ever had acne. Since the skin is an ever living and therefore dying tissue of the body, over a period of time you can slough off the scar tissue and allow new skin tissue to replace it. The only problem here is that the skin underneath must be stimulated to fill in where scar tissue now exists — the RNA-Vitamin E cream is invaluable for this.

SUMMARY

This is the program with precise instructions for the acne patient:

1. Begin with the Liver-Kidney-Bowel Cleansing Fast
2. On the fourth day, as you begin to break your fast add:
    a. 150,000 IU Fish Liver Oil vitamin A
    b. A complete vitamin and mineral supplement. The following can act as a guideline:

SAMPLE FORMULA OF A BALANCED VITAMIN-MINERAL COMPLEX

Vitamin A	25,000IU	Inositol	60mg
Vitamin D	400IU	Folic Acid	400mcg
Vitamin E	400IU	Biotin	100mcg
Vitamin C	1,200mg	Calcium	1000mg
Vitamin B-1	60mg	Magnesium	400mg
Vitamin B-2	60mg	Phosphorus	150mg
Vitamin B-6	60mg	Potassium	99mg
Vitamin B-12	100mcg	Iron	15mg
Niacin	30mg	Iodine	225mcg
Niacinamide	30mg	Copper	2mg
Pantothenic Acid	100mg	Chromium	500mcg
PABA	60mg	Manganese	15mg
Choline	60mg	Zinc	15mg
Selenium	50mg		

c.   Apply a combination adsorbent clay and zinc preparation every morning on arising, leaving it on at least 10 minutes. Remove with a moistened terrycloth wash rag.

d.   Repeat "c" at about 5:30 PM

e.   Apply combination RNA-Vitamin E cream at bedtime and leave on overnight.

f.   Make sure that all refined flour, refined sugar products are eliminated. I suggest following the Creative Restoration Diet.

g.   Physical activity is highly recommended to keep circulation and elimination up to par.

Sounds simple, doesn't it? Well, all I can say is try it and watch your skin clear up. In a few instances, the condition appears to worsen temporarily as the underlying infection comes to the surface. I have suggested the use of the adsorbent application three times daily under these circumstances as this helps draw out the impurities faster.

Chapter 9

BEAUTY THAT DOESN'T RUB OFF AT NIGHT

If it were not for the fact that people have to eat, cosmetics would be the most commonly purchased item in the United States. This search for beauty from the outside should be examined in the light of fact and practical application. There is no way that a beautiful bloom of youth can be restored by something that can be purchased in a bottle. Such applications to simulate color and texture that do not exist are readily apparent upon examination. But this book will not be written in a negative tone. I intend to show you that vitality and life can be restored to your skin which is so often lost as one adds years to his or her life.

Such restoration is not temporary but will endure the sun and wind. Many are of the opinion that famous actresses are constantly going in for face lifts — the facts of the matter are that few actually do. Most of them take time to learn what keeps the skin looking young and then practice that way of living. Since personal beauty is a very special and highly desirable quality from which comes great satisfaction and many rewards, any effort to achieve it can only lead to benefit for anyone who pursues it.

HEALTHY GLOW

Let's talk about that healthy looking glow which associates beauty to most people. What gives the skin a healthy glow is a good supply of red blood flowing near the surface. If you are slightly anemic, the color will be more sallow or pale. The obvious treatment for that is to increase the iron rich food intake or use a supplement which contains iron.

Under some circumstances, the pale appearance may be due to a buildup of dead skin cells on the surface but this can easily be taken care of by the use of a skin exfoliator. These marvelous substances belong to the clay family and with special processing, literally become a "molecular sponge" which lifts off the dead skin cells and allows the new cells underneath to emerge.

Often, poor circulation can be a major factor in preventing that "glow" from showing. Poor circulation can be the result of stress or fear — a good example is the paleness of one who has just heard bad news. Since we live stressful lives as a general rule, we should turn our attention to those factors which might help us to accommodate stress without reacting in a blood vessel constricting way. In general, the B complex vitamins help more than any other, with pantothenic acid, thiamine, vitamin B-12, and PABA being possibly the most important. When these nutrients are deficient, the adrenal glands cannot function to produce the hormones which protect us from the shock of stress.

Let me briefly outline what happens: Stress occurs and the nervous system sends a signal to the adrenals to produce extra adrenalin which will convert an inert storage sugar called glycogen to glucose which is readily available for combination with oxygen to produce energy in the cell. This adrenalin also tightens up the blood vessels temporarily which increases the blood pressure which increases the blood supply to all the tissues of the body, including the face. If certain nutrients, particularly pantothenic acid, are absent, the adrenals are unable to produce its hormones. Another less well known fact is that in the absence of a para amino benzoic acid, another of the B complex family, the liver literally gobbles up these hormones as fast as the adrenals can produce them. We are not sure just why this happens, but it points out the very intricate interdependence of the chemical ingredients of our body. And the basic reason I always suggest that good supplementation consists of a *complete* vitamin and mineral product.

Anyway, your vivacious glow can be affected negatively by your inability to accommodate to stress. Your ability to accommodate to this stress seems to be directly tied into the levels of certain vitamins in your system. So it makes sense to take some precautions in this department.

FOOD SOURCE

I would be the last to insinuate that vitamins are only available from supplemental tablets. Properly cooked foods, in the right combination are of great benefit to your health and certainly to your skin. Foods naturally high in the B complex vitamins, such as whole grain brown rice, fish, nuts, organ meats, poultry, whole grains, cheese, milk and milk products, green leafy vegetables, etc. are very important to include in the daily diet. Be sure that you use as little water in cooking your vegetables as possible, since the cooking water is almost always thrown out, and the water soluble vitamins (which the B Complex are) usually end up in the cooking liquid.

The important vitamins A, D, and E are commonly found in green and yellow fruits and vegetables, milk, milk products, fish, eggs, butter, and organ meats. These are more stable in cooking and do not need as much care, but they do lose much of their vitamin content upon exposure to oxygen and heat, so keep them refrigerated and tightly covered.

ARTERIOSCLEROSIS

A physical condition which can effect your appearance is arteriosclerosis or hardening of the arteries. This condition particularly affects the small capillaries near the surface of the skin which must be filled with blood in order to give you that rosy glow. But even if you do have arteriosclerosis, take heart because there are several things that can be done.

1. Some find that reversing the effects of gravity by lying on an inclined plane — the most common of which is a slant board, will help to open up the capillaries and bring blood to the surface of the skin. An even more drastic, but very effective means, is to stand on your head. This is not as difficult as it may sound. We now have devices which allow you to "stand" on your shoulders without any strain or discomfort to the head.

2. Up until recently, an individual with arteriosclerosis was cautioned not to excise or move too suddenly because of the possibility of a rupture of one of these blood vessels. Now, with the advent of "wholistic" medicine, a few pioneers are advocating a lot of exercise for these patients, on the premise that the increased circulation will bring nutrient chemicals to these areas that are capable of disolving the "hardness." The success rate has been phenomenal and I hope that soon this will be common practice in all doctor's offices.

As far as you are concerned, exercise can only help you — whether you have an arteriosclerosis or not. The biggest deterrent to exercise is that most exercises are boring and the individual soon finds excuses for not doing them. So here are a few tips that may make it easier.

a. Take a minimum of a one-mile walk twice a day at a brisk pace — this can be to the local market or just around the local area.

b. Swimming, tennis, golf, bicycling, etc., are all acceptable, but remember — they must be done on a daily basis if they are a substitue for your walking.

c. A home unit which will accomplish what all these exercises will, in a much shorter time, is now available. This is the mini-trampoline, an ingenious device which can be stored under most beds or in a closet when not in use, but which will restore circulation faster than any means I know. It is safe (models have attachable side rails if you feel uneasy) and gets the job done while you have fun. Five minutes on this is worth 30 minutes or more of rapid walking.

d. Certain vitamins and minerals can help. The arteriosclerotic individual may suffer from a deficiency of oxygen in his or her blood stream. Vitamin E, now rather well known, can be very effective in alleviating this condition. It increases the blood's supply of available oxygen by improving the transportation of oxygen by the red blood cells. It also reduces the need of the heart for oxygen by making the heart become a more efficient pump. And if that isn't enough, vitamin E also acts as a vasodilator, at least of the capillary beds, and improves capillary permeability which is the capacity to permit a better exchange of oxygen and nutrients to enter the cell. So, vitamin E can be one of the most important vitamins for beauty.

The mineral copper, although often not considered, is very essential for the normal flexibility of the arteries in the body. Thus a supplement without copper does not have this very important ingredient that can help deter aging.

THE BEAUTY VITAMINS AND MINERALS

VITAMIN A.   Some cosmetologists have referred to this as "the long life vitamin" and many well-known stage and film star personalities (personally known to me) use high potency vitamin A for youthful, radiant skin. It not only keeps the skin firm by supplying essential nutrients to the layer of fat immediately under the skin which prevents sagging, but also lubricates the skin and prevents dryness. Deficiency signs are dry, rough skin, cracking nails, dry and brittle hair, dandruff. I know how important the appearance of your nails is to you girls; let me assure you that, next to protein, vitamin A is the most important nutrient you can consume to have firm but still flexible nails.

VITAMIN B-1.   This vitamin often helps to serve as a buffer against stress and strain. Fatigue, depression, lack of the joy of living are often traceable to a deficiency of B-1, in fact some doctors are now prescribing B-1 instead of mood altering drugs and getting excellent results. Remember, when you are smiling, it is hard not to be beautiful.

VITAMIN B-2.   An important vitamin for healthy skin and particularly for the eyes. Sparkling eyes can be one of your most recognizable and remembered features, so protect them. Other symptoms of deficiency are cracks in the corner of the mouth, a feeling of sand under the eyelids, sensitivity to light.

VITAMIN B-6.   This vitamin is an important factor in the metabolism of fats and fatty acids so necessary to the health and beauty of your skin. Doctors often refer to it as the anti-dermatitis factor, or a substance which has value in the treatment of skin disorders, dry scalp, and oily skin.

VITAMIN B-12.   Known by almost everyone, this vitamin is famous for its treatment of pernicious anemia. Vitamin B-12 dificiency is most often characterized by both mental and physical dullness. Small amounts bring about miraculous results.

134

NIACIN (Niacinamide). First discovered when the cause of the dread disease pellagra was determined to be a deficiency of niacin in the diet, this vitamin has great effect on the health of the skin. Since the first symptom of pellagra is dermatitis, or inflammation of the skin with blemishes, many scientists are convinced that many of the skin conditions seen today are really the beginnings of pellagra and treat these skin problems with large doses of niacin.

PABA (Para-Amino-Benzoic Acid). Although this nutrient has many other functions, the one most involved with beauty is its use to prevent the graying of the hair of animals. Some claim that they have seen this same effect in humans.

INOSITOL. A vitamin which works hand in glove with vitamin B-6 to make sure that the fatty layer under the skin is properly fed and that excess oils do not pour out on the skin.

CHOLINE. Assists inositol in fat metabolism, and also is a factor in the production of adrenalin, without which your beauty quotient goes down, down, down.

PANTOTHENIC ACID. By far the best known anti-graying vitamin, pantothenic acid is also important for the health of the adrenals, and as a protection against dermatitis.

CALCIUM AND PHOSPHORUS. Dental decay is not a beautiful sight, and we know that such decay can at least be partially be prevented by keeping our stores of these two minerals in plentiful supply. Also, calcium and phosphorus are instrumental in keeping our bones strong which allows for an erect carriage instead of a stooped or slouching position.

IODINE. The thyroid must have iodine to make its hormones. When the thyroid is lacking in function, dry skin, brittle hair, and a tendency toward obesity occurs.

DO I REALLY HAVE TO TAKE EXTRA VITAMINS?

Some have said to me "Do I really have to take extra vitamins? Can't I get all of them in the food I eat?" My answer will always be the same — "Yes" to the first question and "No" to the second. I base some of my enthusiasm for these supplements on a notable statement from Dr. Tom Spies: "The expensive way to use vitamins is to avoid them, develop nutritional failure, and lose your job." I could paraphrase that to read "lose your wife or husband or lover" but the thought is still there and as true today as it was 30 years ago when Dr. Spies uttered it. The other part of my reason is personal experience. I have seen countless hundreds of men, women and children benefitted by the use of nutritional supplements. It is impossible to be benefitted in any way physically or emotionally that does not show in your outward appearance — and that is what beauty is all about. We do not live in the garden of Eden with plentiful, perfect food all about us, just waiting to be picked. We are now living in the age of agribusiness, where the object is to make money without regard for the quality of the food produced. Chemical and other means are used to force growth of vegetables and fruit; tests have shown that you can now buy spinach totally devoid of iron, carrots very low in vitamin A, etc. The use of a good nutritional supplement is the best insurance you will ever buy for your health and beauty.

PROTEIN

The body is composed of many ingredients — water, minerals, vitamins, fat, sugars, and a very complex substance called protein. Every single cell in your body is dependent upon protein for survival. Lack of protein weakens your muscles and makes you flabby. Without adequate protein, your skin begins to sag, shrivel and wither. I cannot put it more succinctly than my departed friend Adelle Davis, "Since your body structure is largely protein, an undersupply can bring about age with depressing speed — muscles lose tone, wrinkles appear, age creeps in; and you, my dear, are going to pot."

This very important stuff also makes up most of your hormones, blood cells, brain, the antibodies which protect you, the enzymes which facilitate so many reactions in the body, and every gland and organ in your body. So it isn't difficult to agree that protein is something to be reckoned with if we wish to maintain our vitality and beauty.

We really do not store much protein in the body; we must have daily intake for maintenance. One fact that is necessary to realize when we consider protein intake is the necessity of digesting or reducing the crude protein foods we eat to their basic ingredients called amino acids. This process of digestion requires enzymes which are made up of proteins, so a vicious circle can occur. A person deficient in protein will have less enzymes to digest any protein which may be consumed. Fortunately, technology has now allowed us to have "predigested" protein available in liquid, powder and tablet form. The advantage of the tablets is that they have no taste while the powder and liquid can be a bit distasteful to some after awhile.

There is often criticism of high protein from some individuals whose philosophy would indicate that the eating of meat and animal related products is esthetically and morally wrong. Others would condemn it on the basis that it is very difficult for the body to process and produces gout, liver and kidney disease, etc. We are not here to engage in such a debate, but I would like to cite the example of the Icelander, the Eskimo and other groups who live in an area where vegetation is practically non-existent. Many studies

137

have indicated that these people have very little, if any, heart disease, gout, liver or kidney disease; even though their diet consists of up to 300 grams of protein per day.

In summary, protein is an absolute must for beautiful skin and contours of the body. One should never forget that protein is the single most plentiful ingedient in his body and must be consumed daily if we wish to keep rejuvenating and regenerating new cells. Digestion of protein is of utmost importance and if any question exists in your mind, it may be wise to consume some predigested protein for your own protection and insurance, or use digestive enzymes with the protein you consume.

RIBONUCLEIC ACID

In his book, "Nucleic Acid Therapy in Aging and Degenerative Disease," Benjamin S. Frank, M.D. describes the formulations by which he believes he has been able to push back the aging process by as much as 12 years or more. His approach is directed not to the symptoms of old age, but to the root cause, to the nucleus of the millions of cells that compose the human body.

Recent research has revealed that the nucleic acid DNA and RNA are cellular components which control heredity and the subsequent ability of the body to keep reproducing its inherited patterns. These strands of amino acids within the cell nucleus govern all life processes in health and disease.

Dr. Frank's work with DNA and RNA and related metabolites demonstrates the importance of these substances, not only to longer life free of disease, but to the wonderful quality of being young as long as you live.

In Dr. Frank's opinion, which seems to have proven out in his clinical experimental work, is that the problem of

138

maintaining youthfulness is really the problem of finding ways to help your body's DNA and RNA renew themselves and keep their patterns of genetic information as clean and fresh as a new etching.

Reduced to its essence, he considers it the problem of supplying the body from external sources with enough viable nucleic acids and with the other nutrients these nucleic acids require to be properly metabolized. Given such nutrition, he believes the nucleic acids themselves stay younger longer, which is reflected in the tissue they reproduce.

The results of his experimental studies provide strong evidence that RNA does indeed visibly reverse aging, especially when given along with other nutrients. Phenomenal results have been achieved by Dr. Frank using a complete dietary regimen rich in nucleic acids. The basic ingredients of the oral formula are RNA (from yeast), amino acids (preferrably predigested), B Complex vitamins, a mineral complex, and lipids or fats.

For both men and women, Dr. Frank also suggests the possibility of using an RNA moisturizing creme externally. He reports, and I can sincerely say that I have also seen the same striking visible effects of the use of such combination therapy. The first effects observed are on the skin of the face. This takes on an aspect of a healthier, rosier looking skin and simultaneously an apparent smoothing of the skin of the face. These effects can occur as early as the first or second week of the combination therapy — external and internal.

After one or two months of treatment, sometimes earlier, there not only is an increase in smoothness and color of the skin, but lines and wrinkles begin to diminish. The first to decrease are the wrinkles in the forehead. The lines around the eyes are next. As the wrinkles decrease there is an increase in skin tightness and an increase in the moistness of the skin as well. These are the advertised but seldom achieved effects of expensive facial creams.

I would like to emphasize that these are only the external visible effects; what is more important is the improvement in general health. I have never seen an individual who did not benefit from a program such as this with better vitality and vigor. Remember that true outward beauty is a reflection of the general physical health.

THE BEAUTY PRODUCTS
THAT DO MORE HARM THAN GOOD

If I can convince you of one thing — don't use soap on your face — I will feel that this will have been worth the effort and you will have benefitted immensely. Let me use an example: Everyone knows that they shouldn't use hand soap to shampoo their hair because it tends to cause dandruff and scaling of the scalp. Why? Because it tends to dry the scalp which produces the characteristic flaking. Why does it produce the dryness? Because by its very nature, soap is alkaline and the application of an alkaline product to the skin destroys the natural protective acid mantle of the skin. Now the body will restore that acid mantle, because the acidity is necessary to destroy bacteria and other contaminants that come in contact with the skin. But if you persist in applying soap to your skin several times a day, the chances of restoring the acid mantle effectively become slim. If you don't use soap, then what do you use to cleanse your face? There are so many products which are effective that space makes it impossible to list them. But I have a personal favorite which is so fabulous that once you start using it, you will never stop. Most people think of this product as a facial mask, but it really is the very best cleanser because it has the physical property of being able to pick up all impurities from the skin without destroying the acid mantle. This product is a clay derivative that has been beneficiated to increase its power of absorption — it literally becomes a "molecular sponge." It is available from your local health food store.

ESTROGEN

The theory which abounded some years ago and is still favored by some today is that the use of estrogen will retard the aging process. No question about it, to some extent this therapy is successful, but the possible price to pay for such indiscriminate use of a powerful drug is something which should not be taken lightly. Modern research has linked the use of estrogen and other related hormone compounds with a demonstrable increase in the incidence of cancer. I do not believe that under any circumstance would I suggest that someone use hormone therapy for controlling the aging process when other means are available which do not produce side effects.

Some women are of the opinion that exercising the facial muscles will create sags or ridges which may become unsightly. This is far from the truth. In the first place the facial musclature is of the type that will not bulge in an unsightly fashion. Secondly, there are two exercises which I have suggested with much success to many women for correction of facial problems. The first is for double chins: Sit in a chair and extend your head backward as far as it will go. Now open and close your mouth in an exaggerated chewing motion, being sure to stretch the muscles under the chin and the front part of your neck. Keep it up until the lower jaw becomes fatigued. As soon as these muscles tone up the double chin, it will pull up and disappear. The second one is for sagging jowls and baggy cheeks. It can be done while you are sitting, standing, lying, or even while driving the car after the children or to the grocery store. Clench your teeth, grimace your mouth as wide as possible, trying to touch your ears with the corner of your lips and say a-a-a-a-r-r-r-gh. This also has some advantage if you are driving in rough traffic, people see you with that terrible, man-eating expression on your face and they will stay out of your way. Anyway, the basic fact remains — exercise is good for your face, just as it is for the rest of your body. It tones up and makes pleasing contours of sagging, loose muscles.

SUMMARY

Age does not have to mean wrinkles, crows feet, sags and bags. There is no reason why you cannot maintain your firmness and tone that was originally intended when your genes determined your general outline. Breakdown of this form is a direct result of an increased state of catabolism or death of cells instead of a state of anabolism or rebirth of new cells as the old die off. You can influence which state your body is in and reap the benefits of an increased feeling of wellbeing as well as seeing the results in the mirror. I have had countless women tell me that they actually look younger than they did five years ago after using the suggestions contained in this booklet. And the proof really comes when someone who hasn't seen you for a few years comes up and says, "I can't believe it's you! You look younger and more beautiful than when I saw you four years ago." The decision is up to you — sure it takes a little work, but all things that are worth having must be earned.

BEAUTY PROGRAM FOR YOU

Many professional motivators use the slogan "Plan your work, then work your plan." You, too, can have a planned program that will certainly be rewarding in the physical benefits you receive and the admiring glances that are thrown your way. I cannot be there to tell you to do it every day, but if you once begin and see the results which will come so quickly, I am sure you will never deviate from the routine that keeps your skin tone up and your figure trim. Your skin is not just an inert covering like the glove you put on your hand. It is a living organ and needs nourishment and exercise like all other organs must to work well. The beauty program which follows is your invitation to a new you!

RSVP ASAP

1. Use a food supplement rich in those ingredients so necessary for a healthy skin. The following would be my recommendation as a broad-spectrum, all-inclusive beauty formula:

Vitamin A	25,000IU
Vitamin D	800IU
Vitamin E	400IU
Vitamin C	1,000mg
Vitamin B-1	50mg
Vitamin B-2	50mg
Vitamin B-6	50mg
Vitamin B-12	50mcg
Niacinamide	50mg
Pantothenic Acid	50mg
Folic Acid	400mcg
Biotin	50mcg
PABA	30mg
Inositol	50mg
Choline	50mg
Calcium	250mg
Phosphorus	50mg
Iodine	150mcg
Iron	10mg
Magnesium	100mg
Copper	2mg
Zinc	10mg
Potassium	66mg
Manganese	20mg

RNA 100mg
Ovarian Substance 100mg
Predigested Protein 1,000mg

2. EXERCISE — Whether you take a brisk one-mile walk twice daily or go dancing, play tennis, swim or whatever, the important thing is to firm up and tone up those muscles. The use of a slant board is excellent for home personal exercises as is the mini trampoline which can give you more exercise in five minutes than most of us can stand.

3. FOOD — Don't neglect taking care in the choice of the food you eat. Be sure it is high in protein, particularly the complete amino acid pattern foods such as fish, cheese, meat, eggs and dairy products. Raw vegetables with lots of fiber are also a must on your table — you may surprise yourself and your family just how good they really taste.

4. RNA — Ribonucleic Acid has been one of the really exciting developments in facial and body skin tone. The use of this substance both externally and internally is beneficial.

5. SOAP — Do not use harsh, alkaline soaps on your face, but instead do use a 'molecular sponge' type clay which will pick up all the impurities without destroying the protective acid mantle on your skin.

6. FACIAL EXERCISE — Don't be afraid to exercise your facial muscles. What you don't use you will lose is an old saying that is very true for muscles — and when muscles begin to atrophy, they sag. Prevent that by using your facial muscles in specific exercises.

It is never too late to start a good thing. Regardless of your physical age, you can start on a rejuvenating program which may apparently turn back your time clock 10 or more years. The new you will add years to your life and life to your years.

Chapter 10

PROSTATE

Thousands of men yearly face the problem of prostatic enlargement, with the symptoms of painful urination, difficult urination, urine retention, infection, and tenderness. As with all disease, we should look at prostatic hypertrophy as abnormal, and not something to expect as we reach 45 or 50 years of age. Statistics would tell us that every fourth man at the age of 52 has prostate problems. If such a disease could be considered normal, then all men should have it at the same approximate time in life — but obviously many escape from it. This booklet will attempt to show you the full picture regarding the prostate and its health — or lack of it.

Because the prostate is removable, and the removal of it does, in fact, cure the symptoms which the individual suffered, very little definitive research has been done on what the causes are — and more important, what can be done to help without operating. Let's examine the prostate so we understand its function and why we men are so often troubled by it.

LOCATION AND FUNCTION

The prostate gland is located very near the opening from the male bladder. It has, literally lying on it, the urethra, a

145

tube used to drain the bladder. When the prostate is enlarged or swollen, the pressure on the urethra interferes with the normal flow of urine. The main function of the prostate is to produce the fluids which act as vehicles for the male sperm. Without these fluids, the male literally becomes sterile, although his libido is usually not affected. On the other hand, the male with prostate problems often has serious problems with his sex life, primarily because of the urine retention situation and possible low grade infection. Another sobering fact regarding the prostate is the high incidence of cancer in this gland. In the female, ovarian, uterine, and breast cancer seem to predominate, but in the male, prostate cancer is the most prevalent among the reproductive organs. This also explains to some extent the willingness of physicians to remove this gland even when minor difficulty is present as a cancer preventive measure.

THE LOWLY PUMPKIN SEED

A well-proven method of prostate enlargement prevention should be a cause for rejoicing among all men who value their health. As with every organ in the body, the prostate is composed of specialized arrangements of amino acids (protein), fatty acids (fats), and minerals. I would like to discuss the fatty acids at this time, most particularly their importance to the proper function of the prostate.

Most of the very important functions in our body are the result of hormones, which are secreted by glands. The hormones need many substances in order that they may be formed by the glands, but among the most important are the fatty acids. If the fatty acids are not present in adequate amounts, hormonal production suffers seriously, as does the function which the hormone triggers. In the case of the prostate, certain doctors have found that the addition of foods high in the fatty acids had a rejuvenating effect on the gland and often kept it functional throughout the entire life of the individual.

Dr. W. L. Cooper, M.D. of Los Angeles conducted an experiment involving nineteen patients to which he gave unsaturated fatty acids as a treatment for prostate problems. No other treatment was given. The results were as follows:

1. All cases showed a lessening of residual urine — that is, urine remaining trapped in the bladder. In 12 of the 19 cases there was no residual urine at the end of the treatment.
2. For 13 of the 19 patients, the treatments ended their getting up at night to urinate.
3. There was a decrease in fatigue and leg pains and an increase in sexual libido in all patients.
4. Cystitis or bladder inflammation cleared up as the residual urine disappeared.
5. Dribbling was eliminated in 18 of the 19 cases.
6. In all cases, the force of the urinary stream was increased.
7. In all cases the size of the prostate gland was rapidly reduced.

Folk medicine in many countries of Europe tells us that the men of Bulgaria, Ukrania, Transylvania (Germany), and Anatolia (Turk) were well aware of the fact that eating a handful of pumpkin seeds daily would prevent prostate problems and thus enhance their virility. When the medical university of Vienna investigated these areas, they found prostatic hypertrophy almost totally non-existent. One of the doctors involved said of the pumpkin seed eating: "This seed has scientifically determined effects on intermediary metabolism; it is regenerative, invigorative, and revitalizing.

There is involved herein a native plant hormone which affects our own hormone production in part by substitution and in part by direct proliferation."

Why should folk lore and folk medicine prescribe the pumpkin seed as the scientific prevention for prostate difficulty and the specific guarantee for male potency? Certainly the function of seeds in carrying the life spark from one generation to the next approximates the function of the reproductive organs in human beings. There seems little doubt that the actual chemical substances that enable the seed to germinate and to produce another plant with the characteristics of the parent are present in reproductive organs of animals — the same hormones, the same enzymes, the same vitamins and minerals. Primitive agricultural people observe, of course, how seeds reproduce and without any knowledge of chemistry, of vitamins, hormones and all the rest, are able to apply the same natural laws to their own health. They believe that eating the part of the plant responsible for reproduction they will enhance their own ability to do the same. Pumpkin seeds are tasty, easy to find, an excellent high protein food, and just may have some properties which will prevent you from having prostate problems — or even assist you in overcoming them if you are now suffering. It seems that a handful or so a day is adequate, but you should do it religiously every single day.

VITAMINS AND CHLOROPHYLL

Many doctors have been very observant in their daily work, and over a period of time associate certain phenomena with certain disease processes. Dr. Benjamin F. Sieve, M.D., Boston, wrote an article on the nutritional prevention of prostate surgery. His theory in general is that

148

vitamins and hormones work together to create health. Infection, emotional upsets and mechanical interference with food intake prevent a proper nutritional state. In studying 200 cases, Dr. Sieve found that infection was one of the specific causes in 60 percent of the cases of prostate hypertrophy. Along with the infection went nutritional deficiency and lack of hormone production. In a study of 100 patients with prostate problems slated for surgery, Dr. Sieve was able to avert surgery by treating them with nutritional therapy in 70 percent of the cases.

Let's examine some of the specific nutritional factors which should be used for infections.

VITAMIN A — Whenever infection is mentioned anywhere in the body, vitamin A should immediately come to mind. In the case of the prostate, vitamin A is particularly indicated because it is heavily lined with mucous cells which absolutely need a plentiful supply of vitamin A to resist or overcome infections. This very essential vitamin does not actually kill germs itself, but, instead, preserves the function of the mucous membrane which is covered with tiny hairs called cilia.

The cilia are in constant motion and trap germs and other foreign matter, sweeping them along the tract for expulsion. When sufficient vitamin A is not present in the system, the cells which produce the cilia are sloughed off, and are replaced by scaly, hard cells.

VITAMIN C — Vitamin C is so important that nature has arranged for most animals to manufacture within their own bodies more of this substance whenever they are exposed to infective type germs. Unfortunately, man is not one of those animals, and must rely upon his intake to furnish whatever vitamin C is necessary. Dr. R. F. Klenner, M.D., enthusiastically states: "Vitamin C, besides being an essential vitamin, is a super antibiotic." If the problem with the prostate is caused by infection 70 percent of the time, doesn't it make good sense to use the body's own infection fighter on a daily basis for prevention and in super amounts if the problem has already developed?

CHLOROPHYLL — Everyone who has taken elementary science is familiar with chlorophyll, the green coloring material in plants. Since the diet of man includes such green plants, and a sick or nutrient deficient plant usually exhibits a gradual loss of color (indicating less chlorophyll), much study has been done on the possible effect of this substance in man. It was first found that it demonstrated a deodorant effect, but this was carried further when the deodorant effect was found to occur because of the detoxifying properties chlorophyll possessed. This systemic detoxifying effect acted as a tonic, useful in most debilitated states associated with chronic disease.

Then it was found that chlorophyll acted as a healing factor, particularly of the mucous membranes where it helped to combat inflammation. Next on the list was the discovery of sex hormone precursors present in this incredible 'blood' of plant life. It was also found to be a source of the fat soluble vitamin factors (A, E, K) and essential fatty acids. Dr. Seive found that the addition of chlorophyll capsules to the diet of his prostate patients was of great help.

From the above, it would seem that chlorophyll is just what the doctor ordered if you have a prostatic problem. It also leads us back to the basic statement that degenerative disease is a lack of adequate food factors in the dietary of man. Look at the diet of the average American male — how much chlorophyll containing foods does he eat on a daily basis?

THE PROSTATE GLAND AND ZINC

Zinc is a bit of a newcomer to the nutritional scene. But it might be wise to consider the fact that the normal prostate gland contains more zinc than any other gland in the entire body. Also that a diseased prostate gland has a very low concentration of zinc. And that, for some reason, vitamin C seems to be more potent as an anti-infective in the presence of zinc. You can draw your own conclusions, but the presence of an adequate amount of zinc in the body certainly would seem to be prerequisite for prostate health.

An interesting sidelight that gives food for thought is the fact that of all the foods available to man, oysters outshine other foods in zinc content by a ratio of about 4 to 1 as compared to its nearest competitor which is wheat germ. And who hasn't heard of the rejuvenative, restorative, aphrodisiac properties of the oyster? Could it be the zinc content? Amazing how often what is considered folklore is proven by research to have sound basis in fact.

THE PROSTATE AND PROTEIN

Since there are often many different ways to accomplish the same end result, we may become confused as to which is the correct or 'only' way. I personally do not believe that such an approach (this is "THE" answer) is possible when dealing with the body. So far, we have discussed pumpkin seeds, vitamins, chlorophyll, and zinc as being important to the health of the prostate gland. Now it is time to look at this gland from a structural view.

The cellular structure of all tissues in the body is made up of a protein membrane or cell wall. The glandular cells are particularly high in their protein content, which makes predatory animals always eat the glandular tissue of their kill first, leaving the muscle meat for the scavengers. Also natives instinctively know that the organ and glandular tissue is of superior food value and the hunters are privileged to consume it, while the women and children get the rest.

Different organs and glands are made up of different ratios of the amino acids, thus giving them their individual characteristics. By accident, two doctors found three amino acids which are very important to the health of the prostate. The physicians were treating a group of allergic patients with a mixture of three amino acids — glycine, alanine and glutamic acid. One of the patients thus treated volunteered the information that his urinary symptoms had disappeared while he took the amino acid mixture. This led to a trial of the same compound on non-allergic patients with urinary symptoms. Patients with enlarged prostates and associated urinary symptoms experienced prompt and rather spectacular relief. They remained free of the symptoms while taking the compound, but often after discontinuing the medication the symptoms returned.

A controlled experiment was set up. A series of 40 cases of prostatic enlargement, previously ascertained to be benign, or non-cancerous, were included. Symptoms of discomfort were present in 35 of the patients, 39 complained of the urge to void often during the night; 23 experienced delayed urination; 29 suffered with excess frequency of urination; and 27 complained of extreme urgency to void which felt uncontrollable. The average age of the patients was 60 years, however their age range was from 37 to 75 years. The average duration of their complaints was 4 years.

The 40 men were divided into two groups. The odd-numbered cases were given glycine-alanine-glutamic acid in supplemental form after each meal for three months. The second group, or even-numbered patients, were also given tablets on the same schedule, except that their tablets did not contain the amino acids, nor any other active ingredient.

Of the men who were treated with the amino acids, the following results were noted:

1. 92% had a diminishing of the size of the swollen prostate.
2. 32% had a complete return to normal size of the prostate.
3. 72% of the patients completely eliminated the need to get up at night to void.
4. 95% of the patients were considerably relieved of the need to get up at night.
5. 81% of the patients reported relief from urgent urination.
6. 73% reported that frequency of urination was noticeably less.
7. 70% indicated that delayed urination was remedied.

There was no comparable improvement in any of the patients who did not receive the amino acids until, after two months, they were switched from the inactive tablets to the amino acid compound.

There were no ill effects whatsoever in any of the patients as a result of the amino acid therapy. It was also noticed that edema, or swelling, of other parts of the body disappeared during treatment. Edema is known to be one of the most important symptoms of protein deficiency. So the conclusion that inadequate protein intake did not furnish the patient with adequate amino acids for healthy prostate tissue makes good sense — just as a diet high in protein would be an excellent protection against the problems presented by a swollen prostate gland.

NUCLEOPROTEINS

While we are on the subject of proteins, we should examine the intricate and very precise way that the body has of reproducing a cell which is worn out and needs to be replaced. Within each cell there is a complex chain of nucleic acids called DNA or deoxyribonucleic acid. This very minute, but complicated, structure has the blueprints for rebuilding the tissue cell when its life cycle has been completed. Under normal circumstances, this rebuilding would take place every 120 days but due to wear and tear, it may occur more often.

With precise knowledge, the DNA will form RNA (ribonucleic acid) and send it out to the blood stream to gather specific amino acids and other building materials to restructure the cell. The body with its infinite wisdom will recycle some of the components of the old cell through the liver for future use and excrete the useless material via the urine. This is all well and good, but sometimes due to circumstances of impaired absorption of nutrients, inadequate dietary, or other factors, the DNA becomes sluggish and does not respond to a signal from the worn out cell for rebuilding. When cells do not rebuild at a rapid enough rate, degenerative disease sets into that area. It loads up with toxic waste products, becomes congested and loses some of its normal function.

Scientists have long been intrigued by the idea that those who used organ or glandular tissue as a part of their diet often seemed to have better organ and glandular health than those who did not. Liver is an excellent example. At one time, the use of raw liver was treatment 'par excellence.' Many used it and received miraculous results. When the chemist tried to substitute the nutrient ingredients found in liver, such as the B Complex, iron, etc., in a separate compound, he found that the results were not the same. The missing ingredient could have been the DNA or a stimulating substance for a particular glandular tissue found only in that gland. This entity seems to be universal in that the use of heart tissue from the cattle family will assist the regeneration of heart tissue in humans. The same holds

154

true for the prostate.

For this reason, I have always used glandular extracts when I felt the glandular structure of a particular individual was sluggish or malfunctioning. Even if the exact mechanism is not known, it works in practice and that is good enough for me.

HOW ABOUT PROSTATIC MASSAGE AND HOT SITZ BATHS?

Prostatic massage and hot sitz baths are time honored remedies and certainly give a certain amount of relief. I have to compare them with giving two aspirin to the man who has his finger jammed in the door. He may be relieved of the major portion of pain, but you haven't solved the cause of the problem yet. Their use with the nutritional program outlined will certainly enhance the recovery, but I do not recommend their use alone if you wish to overcome the basic problem.

PROGRAM FOR PROSTATIC HYPERTROPHY

1. Follow the Creative Restoration Diet outlined at end of this book.
2. Eat a handful of pumpkin seeds every day.
3. Use a least 3,000 mg. vitamin C daily.
4. Use at least 50,000 IU vitamin A daily.
5. Chlorophyll capsules — about 2 daily.
6. Zinc — at least 30 mg. daily.
7. The three amino acids — glycine, alanine, and glutamic acid — are most plentifully found in casein, the protein of milk. Use some daily.
8. Nucleoprotein concentrate of prostate — about 2 daily.

155

The above program will help support the vital rebuilding and regenerative processes in the body. They should not be considered as medicines but as special foods with special effects on the body. They are readily available from your health food stores and are a sensible approach to a difficult but common problem.

Chapter 11

CANCER: CAUSE AND CONTROL

Cancer is a hideous, double-headed monster. In its beginning, it grows silently and stealthily, with scarcely a ripple made in what is apparently normal physiology and metabolism. The first sign may not be a visible tumor, but instead a feeling of lethargy, weakness and weight loss, not reflected in the normal blood panels. Indeed, a symptom pattern which is practically universal is the increasing weakness and lethargy without any apparent reason.

A disturbance in liver enzymes and blood count is too often a late phenomenon in cancer, and the diagnosis is thus also late.

Let us go back to the primary cause of cancer. Certain factors are always present, for cancer grows in the sterile fields of malnutrition. The work of Drs. Virginia Livingston, Eleanor Jackson, *et al.*, in various clinics and laboratories around the country has incriminated a specific organism similar to the tuberculosis mycobacterium. This has been designated the Progenitor Cryptocides. This organism is always present and is a factor in the beginning phases of cancer. It has been seen in numerous laboratories but always considered heretofore as a contaminant.

However, the blood of cancer patients is always swarming with these organisms which can be cultured. Animals injected with the blood or fluid from cancer patients will develop cancer and, in turn, this can be transmitted to other experimental animals. The organism is present everywhere and tenacious in its characteristics. But it cannot flourish where there is normal metabolism.

The work of Nobel Prize winner, Dr. Otto Warburg, has proven that normal cells can become cancerous wherever there is a decrease in the oxygen tension and a disturbed metabolism. The organism, Progenitor Cryptocides, hereafter designated P.C., first produces a large number of bacteria in the blood, which later become a fulminating and deadly toxic state when the conditions are right. In one phase of life cycle, it exists as a virus-like organism, and as such can penetrate through the walls of an abnormal diseased or weakened cell; set up housekeeping in the nucleus and distort the genetic code, symbolized by its DNA and RNA, and the cell becomes an abnormal cell which can only produce further abnormal cells. Or it may actually destroy the cell and where one virus penetrated the nucleus, many are produced by reproduction, using the cell as its nutrient source. The organism in its mature form can be seen as a cannibalizing parasite destroying the red blood cells and other normal cells of the body.

PRESENT STATUS OF CANCER THERAPY

In an article taken from *the Medical World News* of October 3, 1977, entitled "Cancer Survival: Uphill Slowly," it states that up to 1973 the five year survival rates show "remarkably little improvement over the past quarter of a century despite countless presumed advances in diagnosis, treatment, and availability of care." That is the dismal reality disclosed in a National Cancer Institute report titled "Cancer Patient Survival." This article reveals that there has only been a 1%-2% improvement in survival rates in cancer of uterus, breast, bladder, prostate, cervix, colon,

158

rectum, stomach, lung and pancreas since 1950. This is an amazing confession coming from the "Delphian Oracle" of medical orthodoxy.

We can put a man on the moon; we can do cardiac transplants and have the patient survive a few months. We can do remarkable feats of coronary bypass surgery, but with all the exquisite and sophisticated armament at our fingertips, very little progress has been made in cancer survival, and none where metastases has occurred. Why this serious lack of results? First, medical science is treating a disease which is almost a total mystery to them. At this date the average M.D. has no concept as to the cause, let alone a successful treatment.

There are two phases to this double-headed monster's existence: One is the invasion of the blood and lymphatic system, in which there is an actual multiplication of bacteria in the blood and in the later stages, an explosive toxemia. The other stage is when the normal cells of the body which have been degraded in their function are invaded by the virus-like phase of the Progenitor Cryptocides. The cell, then, will either be destroyed or become mutated from its aberrant genetic code and can then only produce abnormal cells. This multiplication of cells without the control of the normal body enzymes is the phase of abnormal new growth that we know as cancer. Rapid multiplication into surrounding areas is called metastasis.

FORMULA

We can present the factors contributing to the phenomena of abnormal new growth as follows: the formula may be expressed as X + S + T +MC + H = Cancer. To break this down, X represents the specific organism always present, the Progenitor Cryptocides; S represents Stress; T represents Toxemia; MC represents the Malnourished Cell; H represents Hereditary Factors. If we can change, modify, or eliminate any factor on the left side of the equation, we can of course reduce the incidence of cancer. Since there are many factors present which contribute to the cancer syndrome, the treatment is multipurpose and holistic; a concept totally foreign to orthodoxy today. The tumor mass is a late symptom and often signals the terminal phase of cancer. The pathological signs are specific for each organ or area involved but this does not mean that a specific treatment is needed for each area involved, for instance collagen tissue, bone marrow, skin, internal organs, lymphatic tissue, etc.

Medicine is preoccupied with the study of abnormal or dead cells. Investigation must begin with careful dark field microscopic studies of living blood fluid; for example the urine, feces, blood, etc. Elimination of the focus (tumor mass) is futile without removal of toxemia, stress, malnourishment, etc. The first objective should be to detoxify and then rectify. This involves removal of stress, correction of dietary deficiencies, chelation, megavitamin-mineral therapy, and immunology. There is a place for surgery, radiation and chemotherapy, but we feel they are all over-utilized.

A good example of the holistic approach to carcinoma is in the work being done at the famous Jankers Clinic in Bonn, Germany. In this clinic they use surgery judiciously, radiotherapy selectively, and also chemotherapy when specifically indicated. However, they endeavor to combine these therapies with a holistic approach, which emphasizes good basic nutrition, and they have recently begun to use a combination of proteolytic enzymes and the vitamin A therapy.

160

PROTEOLYTIC ENZYMES

The specific enzymes they use with great effectiveness is the Wobe-Mugos manufactured by a company in Munich, Germany. These enzymes contain beef pancreas, calf thymus, papaya, bromelin, and several other extracts. They have the ability to dissolve cancer cells selectively in tissue cultures which is an index to what occurs in the living body. These enzymes have been injected directly into the tumor mass, causing cell death without invading the borders of the surrounding health tissue. They have a very satisfying statistical reduction in the frequency of metastases and in the relapse rate. There is also a dramatic improvement in the well-being of the patient, including increased radiation tolerance.

The present work stems from the original research carried on about 50 years ago by Drs. Freund and Karminer. These men observed that cancer cells were dissolved in the test tube when treated with serum of healthy persons. Conversely, if the serum of cancer patients was used, destruction of the tumor cells did not occur. It was postulated that certain proteolytic enzymes in the serum are responsible for the destruction of malignant cells. The serum of healthy persons does possess a higher proteolytic activity than those with carcinoma. Extensive animal experiments have been carried out on the rabbit, rat, and the mouse. The results have been extremely gratifying. In certain clinics, such as the Jankers Clinic of Bonn, such serums are used in the treatment of human carcinoma with a high degree of success.

We should combine the whole program of detoxification and megavitamins with large doses of the proteolytic enzymes, vitamin A, chelated minerals, etc., the surgical removal of tumor masses where they are accessible,

radiation for certain highly sensitive tumors and chemotherapy used very carefully and judiciously in the early
treatment of certain types of leukemias, chorionic car-
cinomas, etc. This holistic approach is meeting with a larger
degree of success than in most clinics in America.
Interestingly enough, there is no incompatibility between
the use of these highly effective proteolytic enzymes,
vitamin A, the whole nutritional program, and the usual
standard orthodox treatments. However, to be most
effective, the holistic approach must be instituted immediately and not as an aftermath to extensive radiation and
chemotherapy. Both of these latter modalities destroy the
body's immune forces and while they will kill a certain
amount of tumor cells, they also are destructive to a large
number of healthy, normal cells. I am confident that this
approach will eventually be accepted by orthodox medicine.
We are also cognizant of the fact that there is a therapeutic
lag sometimes extending over a period of decades between
the discovery of effective treatment and the full acceptance
and utilization of such treatment.

OTHER FACTORS

We might mention some of the famous researchers who
have made a unique contribution in the field of degenerative
diseases, immunotherapy, reversal of the aging process,
prolongation of life, etc. We think first of all of Pasteur and
the Drs. Koch-Robert and later his nephew William Koch, Dr.
Szent-Gyorgi, Dr. Pauling and Dr. Ivy, Dr. Virginia Livingston Wheeler, also Drs. Burkett, Bittner, Rouse, Glover,
etc. Almost all of these physicians have met ridicule,
antipathy and open opposition from their colleagues, and
yet it is impossible to stop the wheels of progress indefinitely. The late, great statesman, Sir Winston Churchill

once said that the tragedy of the human race is that they learn nothing from history. Certainly in the field of healing arts there is no place for pride or prejudice, indifference or opposition to truth.

Consider also the effectiveness of megavitamin therapy in many of the degenerative diseases. Dr. Abram Hoffer of Canada and his colleagues have proven conclusively in thousands of cases that large doses of Niacin, vitamin C and B-6 can help in the rehabilitation of the schizophrenic patient.

Good nutrition is absolutely essential for all degenerative diseases and for the recovery of all illnesses, and yet the average doctor is fed with propaganda to the point that he actually believes that the American diet as used by the majority of the population is adequate for all nutritional needs.

IMMUNE SYSTEM

Without a competent immune system no one recovers from cancer and so we would like to allude briefly to immunotherapy. Such therapy boosts the ability of the body to resist changes from normal — including, but not limited to, cancer.

1. We have a non-specific immunotherapy with BCG, a vaccine against the tubercle bacillus with a history of producing remissions of melanoma, an almost universally fatal form of cancer.
2. We have the active specific immunotherapy in the application of the autogenous vaccine, a substance made from our own fluids that is then re-injected to stimulate antibody response.
3. We have a passive immunity as emphasized by Dr.

Andrew Ivy.

4. We have adaptive immunotherapy by the use of concentrated lymphoid cells and immune RNA.

All of these factors can be utilized by the physician in assisting the body to resist invasion of bacteria and reducing the mutation of cells which produces cancer.

These things have been known for years, and yet organized medicine is very slow in accepting these modalities. There is a serious therapeutic lag from the time a discovery is made until it is utilized. A prime example is Penicillin which lay on the shelf for 14 years after it was discovered by Sir Alexander Fleming. In the interim probably millions of lives were lost that could have been saved. Another example is Pangamic Acid, or B15, first synthesized by Krebs and Krebs in 1951. Later, over ten foreign countries have substantiated its usefulness, and yet it is not officially available in the United States.

RECAP

Let us briefly reconsider some of the factors we have discussed.

1. Progenitor Cryptocides — The PC organism is the agent which is always present in cancer, and yet our emphasis should not be on merely the destruction of this organism. The treatment of cancer is total warfare!
2. Detoxification — Later in this book, we will outline the Liver-Kidney-Bowel Cleansing Fast which we feel is so important in the beginning of any successful attack on a serious disease in the body.
3. Specific Enzymes — Extensive clinical research has indicated that particular enzymes containing pancre-

164

atic enzymes, factors from thymus gland, extracts of papaya and pineapple, and others are effective in actually dissolving cancer cells.

4. Super Nutrition — High dosages of both vitamin A and vitamin C have been proven to have life-extending and tumor-reduction effect. Emphasis on these two nutrients should not take our attention away from a good diet and broad spectrum supplementation with vitamins and minerals.

5. Laetrile, Carcolin, etc. — These unorthodox treatments have one basic factor in their favor — many individuals have found they were effective in their particular case and have visible proof of it. More and more individual states are allowing the use of these formerly prohibited substances. Doctors may now use them without fear of prosecution.

6. Immunotherapy — Judicious use of this form of therapy can often stimulate the body to perform its functions of defense against invading organisms more efficiently.

7. As a final measure, radiation, chemotherapy and surgery may be used to slow down growth, or to remove a tumor in a critical area, but it should be emphasized that the other measures listed above should be used first.

GERSON TREATMENT

The outstanding authority in the treatment of cancer and other allied degenerative diseases was Dr. Max Gerson. This brilliant clinician probably had greater success than any other physician of his time in treating the serious deficiency diseases. He demonstrated that one of the prime causes of cancer was a lack of potassium and a surplus of sodium. He showed that surgery, radiation and chemo-therapy do not restore the normal functions of the entire system in the cancer patient, but are all toxic, damaging and cause stress.

Accoring to Dr. Gerson, the beginning of all chronic disease is the loss of potassium in the cells and bringing in of sodium into the cells. Cancer patients are almost always low in potassium. This upsets the delicate mineral balance of the body, which in turn, affects the cell, allowing less oxygen to enter the cell and less waste products to leave the cell. These cells become malnourished and are wide open to the encroachment of bacteria, and eventually disease — both acute and chronic. Early signs of this process include the swelling, or edema, of the ankles, hands and other areas of the body.

The process of detoxification means the re-introduction into the system of large amounts of potassium. This is accomplished by fresh fruit and vegetable juices. This also helps in the rejuvenation of the liver. The body has all of the inbuilt specific systems to activate enzymes, to inactivate toxic substances and to restore healing. Whether the disease is tuberculosis, multiple sclerosis, arthritis, hepatitis, cirrhosis of the liver, or cancer, the body can perform miracles of healing, providing a system of detoxifi-cation and re-establishment of normal nutrition is carried out.

COFFEE ENEMAS

One of the principal and effective means of detoxifying the body is coffee enemas. Caffeine is recognized by the liver as a poison. It causes a dilation of the bile ducts. There is a vigorous purging effect and large amounts of stagnant bile and toxins are eliminated through the bowel. Now the interesting thing is that when the healing mechanism of the body is being re-activated, the healing is not done selectively but it affects the whole body. So a person with cancer who is being detoxified and is undergoing a healing process will also find very frequently relief from his diabetes, arthritis, chronic skin conditions, epilepsy, and so forth. In the case of diabetes there is often a remarkable reduction in the amount of insulin needed and even a complete reversal of the disease when proper regeneration is carried out. There is no way under heaven that this can be done without proper nutrition, without obedience to all of the laws of health, without proper detoxification and the use of supplements in adequate, or even megadose, amounts.

MINERAL FACTORS

Most of the vitamin preparations on the market today contain minerals but a careful reading of the labels will show that often the vitamins are minimal or in inadequate quantities and the minerals are not in form that is usually utilized by the body. Dr. Hans Neiper of Germany has done extensive work with mineral transporters. In the late 1950s, it was discovered that the cells of the female breast became malignant when there was a loss of magnesium. At the same time, Dr. Hans Selye showed that mild heart cell aging could be prevented with the help of potassium and magnesium chloride. Dr. Neiper found that Aspartic Acid and Orotic Acid, when combined with essential minerals, acted as transporters through the outer cell membrane and the mineral was then made available to the metabolism of the cell.

In Germany and other countries the chelated minerals are in wide use. For instance, the Calcium Orotate has no side effects and is one of the most valuable treatments of osteoporosis and arthritis. Zinc Orotate has been valuable

167

in the treatment of diabetes. In cardiology, Potassium-Magnesium-Aspartate plays a very important role in the management of metabolic heart disease. According to Dr. Neiper, Potassium-Magnesium-Aspartate decreases the death rate from cardiac blockage by an astounding 84%. Magnesium Orotate helps prevent cell death and so does Potassium Orotate. They found a 94% success rate in the treatment of Arteriosclerosis with Magnesium Orotate. These chelated minerals are absolutely essential to health and where there is a deficiency in potassium, magnesium, calcium or other vital minerals, degeneration and necrosis occur. Since cancer is one of the major degenerative diseases that we are faced with, it is logical to think that these chelated minerals which stimulate cell metabolism and prevent early cell aging and death will also be effective in the treatment and control of cancer. It has been shown that the application of active calcium carriers is playing an enormous and significant role in the treatment and management of immune disease. These mineral transporters release the important ions at a site where they are most needed, and this results in the activation of enzymes or restores the structures of the cells by sealing against potential agression. They are simple, harmless, nontoxic, but extremely active in principle.

We should point out that the body normally chelates its minerals with a process known as amino acid chelation and this process is carried out without any effort on our part. A problem occurs when disease is present, or when we do not eat total and complete proteins to furnish the body with the amino acids necessary to carry out the function of chelation, or when an inadequate supply of minerals is included in the diet. Another factor must also be present — hydrochloric acid in the stomach is required for both the breakdown of the protein and the mineral to their basic form. Amino acid chelated minerals are available from your local health food store.

ARE YOU RANCID?

From middle age onward the body ages rapidly. Variations on this theme occur of course, depending on biological individuality.

Many factors, such as heredity, freedom from undue stress and disease and proper nutrition are involved. With age there is an increase in the production of the free radical of super-oxide. These toxic groups unite with fatty tissues or lipids causing rancidity, and starting a chain reaction of degeneration and disease.

Vitamins C and E, and the trace mineral Selenium, act as superoxide scavengers and halt or slow down this process. Vitamin A to a lesser extent is also an anti-oxidant. Oxidation may be compared to the rusting of a nail. Rusty or rancid bodies are more susceptible to disease.

In a recent issue of a prestigious and widely published periodical, *Modern Medicine,* of October 30, 1978, appears this statement: "Dietary habits may contribute to as many as 40% of American cancer deaths," physicians reported at a recent nutritional conference sponsored by the National Cancer Institute and the American Cancer Society. Dr. Earnest Wynder, President of the American Health Foundation, estimates that excessive meat, calorie and fat ingestion, combined with food additives and agricultural chemical residues account for half of all cancer in men and one third of those in women.

It is well known that deep fried foods, barbecued fat, etc., are carcinogenic. So at long last the medical profession is beginning to realize that nutrition has a very valuable part in prevention of disease, particularly cancer and other generative diseases. Years ago, we stated from the podium and in writing that no effective therapeutic bullet would ever be found for the treatment of cancer that does violence to the body's natural defenses in the treatment of that cancer.

In the interim, honest researchers world-wide have diligently sought for a lethal weapon against cancer which would not destroy the normal cells and ruin natural immunity.

Such a substance has been found and when combined with super nutrition, temperance, detoxification, etc., holds a great promise, not only for cancer but for arthritis, hypertension, diabetes, cirrhosis of the liver, etc.

Providentially, a manuscript of enormous importance came to our attention recently. After reading only a few paragraphs we realized that here at last was what we had been searching for most of our professional lives, "a substance, non-toxic in proper amounts, that was effective in treating many degenerative diseases." Like a hungry, tattered beachcomber who had stumbled upon a buried treasure, we felt that here was the answer to many problems. Let me explain.

GERMANIUM

For thousands of years the wise men of the Orient had been extolling the virtues of certain herbs such as Ginseng, certain types of mushrooms, garlic, bamboo sprouts, etc., as a practical answer to many of the current diseases. They had no knowledge of biochemistry or atomic energy which would explain these qualities, but they knew from experience their virtue. Germanium, atomic #32, was discovered by the German chemist Winkler, although its presence as an element was found hypothetically a decade previously by the Russian scientist Mendeleev, proponent of the periodic chart. For 60 years following this, it was largely ignored, and considered a rare element of no particular value.

In 1948, because of its value as a semi-conducting material, it began to be used in transistors and diodes.

170

Germanium appears as a metal but without metallic properties. It was not until the advent of quantum physics that the importance of atomic and molecular electron effects were appreciated. Since all living organisms come under the same laws governing matter, it was hypothesized that man is an aggregate of ultramicroscopic electrical impulses and would respond to the energy exchange in a positive manner. It is also known that excessive hydrogen ions which are positively charged are toxic to the body, acting like dust in a very sensitive machinery; either the hydrogen has to combine with oxygen, forming water and then excreted, or it will be desensitized by the atomic particles of negative ions contained in such substances as germanium. This will act as a detoxifying or inactivating agent.

These ultra-microscopic electrical particles and their qualities in human beings is not surprising when we realize and understand the terms of quantum theory of physics that the human body is merely an aggregate of ultra-minute, electrically charged particles. Then we can understand a little more the specific and important cause and effect of germanium in establishing or maintaining health.

Plants containing large quantities of germanium are without exception those valued as medical herbs in the Orient. We mentioned previously Ginseng, the forest Shelf Fungus, a type of mushroom; the Japanese Shitake mushroom, and the popular mushrooms used in this country are rich in sources of germanium. Germanium greatly enhances the effectiveness of oxygen in body metabolism. All chronic diseases are associated with a lack of available oxygen in body cells. Chronic or sustained oxygen depression (anoxia) always results in degenerative disease and eventually death. The fascinating crystals of germanium, a silver-gray substance, can be more valuable than diamonds, and indeed might be considered the gem of life. Their beauty and value is intrinsic and not merely a glittering jewel to be worn on someone's finger. By enhancing oxygen use, it gives life to deprived cells, allowing more vibrant life.

Dr. Kazuhiko Asai was born in 1908 in a province of Manchuria. He grew up and attended technical institutions in Berlin and in Japan and in 1945 established the Coal Research Institute. The following information has been gleaned from his very important manuscript called "Organic Germanium — A Medical Godsend." At the present time he is carrying on his research work in Tokyo, Japan, in conjunction with a number of medical doctors.

After years of studying germanium, he received very little credit or attention and gradually became incapacitated because of a serious arthritis condition. He was unable to carry on his work and to find the funds necessary to prove his thesis of the value of germanium.

For all appearances germanium is a metal, but it is completely without metallic properties. Its value lies in its ability to act as a semi-conductor. It is an invaluable trace element which does not accumulate in the body; in fact, it is very useful in detoxifying or removing heavy metallic particles such as lead, cadmium, and mercury from the body. Dr. Asai tells of his great discouragement in his incapacity and also mentions the fact that when he was at the very height of his illness he was determined not to give in, but wrote these words in his diary: "I am not going to put forth an argument to justify this loss, nor am I going to surround myself with the feeling of pathos either. I am merely at a loss as to where in a capitalistic, profit-centered society like ours, a person who has set out to do a work of useful nature can find an axis to coordinate his spirit."

It was about this time, on November, 1967, that the last remaining member of his research staff walked into his bedroom holding a test tube of white powder. Raising it slowly, and with an expression on his face which radiated the whole room, he uttered the words Dr. Asai had been waiting ten years to hear: "The water soluble organic germanium compound has at last been synthesized."

Dr. Asai, after acquainting himself with the properties of the valuable element by using it experimentally on animals, was convinced that it had very active healing properties and recalled the words of Einstein, "The perception of mystery is a source of every learning and discovery."With these thoughts he determined to try this material on himself first.

After taking germanium for several weeks, he found to his gratification, that the symptoms of his arthritis were leaving him and he was able once again to resume his laboratory duties. Further studies demonstrated that this substance was effective in degenerative diseases such as diabetes, hypertension, cirrhosis of the liver, epilepsy, and even cancer.

Dr. Asai and his co-laborers demonstrated, in a series of research projects on mice which were injected with cancer cells and would inevitably have developed cancer, that germanium had a cancer inhibiting effect. All the mice which had been placed on the germanium compound survived, while their litter mates who did not receive germanium developed fatal cancer. This test was repeated several times for verification of the results.

It was also demonstrated in the clinic where patients were treated for a variety of disorders that marked improvement of uterine, breast, bladder, prostatic, and pancreatic cancers was attainable.

Dr. Asai stated that the patient taking large doses of organic germanium may feel a certain warmth surging through the body within ten minutes. The yawning ceases, blood becomes less viscous, and the complexion takes on a healthy glow. The patient may be convinced that the material that he has swallowed contains alcohol. However, the healing process begins and is carried on progressively until the patient in so many cases is restored to health. The work of Dr. Otto Warburg of Germany a Nobel Prize winner, showed that the growth of cancer cells is due primarily to oxygen deficiency. Since the cells of our body live in the presence of oxygen, an insufficient supply of oxygen alters the strutures of these cells. He proved in his laboratory experiments that normal cells can become abnormal cancer cells if they are raised in an atmosphere of oxygen deprivation. The dangers of oxygen deficiency in the human body cannot be over-emphasized. Also, the major causes of oxygen deficiency such as smoking, industrial pollutants, and so forth, must be eliminated as far as possible.

Not only is it important to increase oxygen absorption and utilization, it is also important that the positive hydrogen ions which are useless to the body, and which may be compared to dust clogging a delicate machine, be removed by a combination with oxygen and subsequently the formation of water.

To summarize: when we can restore the circulation of normal, well-oxygenated blood carrying sufficient vitamins, minerals and nutrients to the cells, we have accomplished the first stage in reversal of all degenerative diseases. A pure and healthy blood stream is absolutely essential in the treatment of cancer. It is impossible to have a healthy blood stream with a diseased liver, and it is impossible to have a healthy liver with a stagnant, toxic colon. So the treatment of cancer is the treatment of the whole individual. There is a place, of course, for surgery or careful and selective radiation, and at times and in certain forms of extremely malignant and fulminating cancers, the extremely careful use of chemotherapy. None of these modalities are effective in restoring health. They are merely suppresive and at times help to take a load off the natural immune system of the body. Cancer is becoming epidemic and even pandemic. We are impelled to state that it is important to take a sharp, critical look at the present forms of therapy and it is absolutely essential to adopt a natural approach to the problem, which means, in essence, detoxification, the restoration of the body's immune mechanism, and proper nutrition.

Chapter 12

CHOLESTEROL

Let me begin this particular subject with the following statement: "The cholesterol-heart attack cause and effect relationship concept is the most unscientific accepted theory promoted in the past many years."

The mere mention of the word "cholesterol" is enough to strike terror in the hearts of many. It is probably the most commonly misunderstood of the substances which appear normally in the body. Let us list just a few of the body functions of cholesterol:

1. Is a constituent of pituitary, adrenal and gonadal hormones.
2. Is converted to vitamin D upon exposure to ultraviolet light from the sun.
3. Acts as a conductor of nerve impulses.
4. Is present in every body cell and helps to regulate the exchange of nutrients and waste products across the cell membrane.
5. Is a constituent of bile, necessary to emulsify fats.

The following facts can lead to a more rational approach to the whole cholesterol problem:

1. The less cholesterol you take in with your foods, the more your body produces.
2. The more cholesterol you take in with your foods, the less your body produces.
3. The greatest rise in serum cholesterol occurs after the ingestion of excessive carbohydrates and not fat.

The restriction of cholesterol containing foods, such as butter and eggs, actually has very little to do with your cholesterol level. Certain religious orders, whose beliefs insure a complete vegetarian diet, have about the same level of high and low cholesterol readings as the average meat eating individuals. Studies in certain primitive tribes who consume large, even huge, amounts of cholesterol in their normal dietary registered very low serum cholesterol levels. Other studies of individuals who had high cholesterol levels and were put on a very restricted cholesterol intake, demonstrated that for every 100 units of cholesterol removed from the diet, the level in the blood falls by only 3 units. What all this really tells us is that there is no direct relationship on a sound, scientific basis between cholesterol intake and cholesterol levels in the blood.

CHOLESTEROL AND ATHEROSCLEROSIS

Well, if dietary intake of cholesterol doesn't raise cholesterol, then what does? It is an established fact that cholesterol is present in blood vessel disease such as atherosclerosis — what, if any, significance does it have? First of all, I would like to present some facts for your reflection:

1. The atheromatous plaques found on the wall of the artery in atherosclerosis contains not only cholesterol, but fibrin, collagen protein, minerals, triglycerides and phospho-

lipids plus other cementing cells which hold the whole thing together. Why was cholesterol singled out as the villain?

2. Blood cholesterol levels are almost identical for men and women, yet the coronary heart disease rate is much higher for men.

3. Blood cholesterol levels do not continue to increase by any appreciable amounts after the age of 50, but the rate of coronary heart disease increases greatly.

4. A very well controlled study, in which all of the patients had high cholesterol levels, revealed that when the group was divided and 50% had their blood cholesterol levels reduced by medication, the rate of heart disease remained the same for both. Eighteen of each group had serious atherosclerotic problems, even though one group had a 'normal' cholesterol level.

What facts such as the above prove is that a scientific relationship between the levels of blood cholesterol and blood vessel disease is not proven. There are too many variables to consider, and just because it is rather easy to measure blood cholesterol and often find it elevated, no license is given to draw a conclusion. This would be similar to a situation where you were a shopper in a store which was robbed. Since you were there, the conclusion could be drawn that you were the robber. Not so! you cry indignantly, many others were there also.

Again consider this fact: The atheromatous plaque found on the wall of the artery in atherosclerosis, when first formed, contains no cholesterol at all! Fibrin seems to be the first present, after which collagen protein, minerals, cholesterol, triglycerides and phopholipids plus other cementing cells group together to form the plaque. *Why was cholesterol singled out as the villain?*

OTHER STUDIES

1. Contrasts in death rates from heart disease in

countries where fat consumption is the same: The United States, the United Kingdom, and Sweden consume nearly identical percentages of total fat and nearly identical ratios of polyunsaturated fatty acids — yet the death rate from coronary heart disease in the U.S. is three times as high as that of Sweden, and almost two times as high as the rate in the United Kingdom.

2. The Baylor University research study of patients hospitalized for surgical treatment of atherosclerosis: Dr. Michael DeBakey and his research team studied 1,700 patients hospitalized for surgical treatment of atherosclerosis due to its severity. Eight out of ten of these patients had cholesterol levels within the normal average for Americans! Only 20% had a clinically elevated blood cholesterol.

3. The Harvard University study of the effect of exercise on blood cholesterol levels: In a research project, blood cholesterol levels did not rise in healthy young medical students placed on an extremely high-caloric diet with large amounts of saturated fats when the students *increased their physical activity enough to maintain their body weight.* But when they did not exercise while on this same diet, their blood cholesterol levels rose along with their body weight.

4. The Israel study by Brunner: This covered the frequency of heart disease in 5,279 men and 5,229 women, aged 40 to 64, living in collective settlements under uniform environmental conditions. Angina pectoris, blood vessel disease and deaths from heart disease were *2.5 to 4 times higher* in sedentary workers than in physically active workers. In a 6-year follow-up study of 233 men and 40 women, 40 to 64 years old, after their first heart attacks, Brunner found that the deaths in the first 4 weeks were 4.2 per cent for active workers and 22.6 per cent for clerks and office workers — *over 5 times as great!* The total number of deaths 6 years after the first attack was 23.1 per cent in active workers and 54 to 59 per cent in clerks, merchants, and professionals — *over 2½ times as great!*

5. The 10-year Evans County, Georgia, study by Dr. C. G. Hames and his associates: This covered all persons age 40 to 74 in the county and a random 50 per cent of those aged 15 to 39. The results: Coronary heart disease was 8 times as prevalent among white males as black males; but white laborers and small farmers had the same low rate of heart disease as the blacks (thus ruling out racial differences). The great excess of heart disease in the whites was found among the prosperous business and professionals, and large farm owners — groups far more physically inactive than the laborers and small farmers. The amount of animal fat that poor white laborers and blacks ate was vastly higher than that eaten by the more prosperous classes. In fact, pork and pork fat were the mainstay of their diets — the very reverse of what would be expected if fat intake were the cause of coronary blood vessel disease. Even more significant, whether the prosperous groups had high or low blood cholesterold levels, their excess rate of heart disease persisted . . . *thus eliminating the cholesterol level as a factor of importance.* One, and only one factor, correlated with the incidence of coronary heart disease in this tudy, *lack of physical exercise.*

6. The Ireland-Boston Heart Study: (a cooperative research project of Harvard University and the Trinity School of Medicine in Dublin). Its purpose: to rule out heredity factors in the onset of heart disease by studying only blood brothers. Over 600 Irishmen between the ages of 30 and 60 years who have lived in Boston for 10 or more years and their brothers who have never left the old country. The result: The Irish brothers eat 500 calories more a day and almost twice as much butter and eggs as their American brothers (averaging a pound of butter and 14 to 18 eggs a week). Despite this, they weigh 15 per cent less, have lower cholesterol levels and (very important) high blood pressure is less than half as common in the Irish as in their Boston brothers. Why the great difference? Apparently the *greater physical exercise from walking and bicycling that the Irish indulge in daily.*

7. Dr. Paul Dudley White and his associates' study of Harvard athletes: The health records of 355 former Harvard varsity football players (covering the years between 1900 and 1930) were compared for those still living without heart disease and those, living or dead, who developed artery disease. The result: "Those living or dead who developed artery disease habitually took less exercise than those who did not develop it; and no individual in this study who maintained a heavy exercise schedule happened to develop coronary blood vessel disease."

8. The studies of Dr. G. V. Mann and associates of the pastoral Masai tribe of Tanzania in Africa: This tribe lives almost entirely on meat and milk — an extremely high saturated fat diet. Despite this, a clinical survey of 400 Masai men showed them almost free of coronary artery disease at any age. Even blood pressure showed only a slight tendency to increase with age. The blood cholesterol levels were startlingly lower than that of the U.S. population — averaging only 120 mgs. %.

Dr. Mann reports: "The Masai men spend much of their lives as boys walking with the herds. As warriors they are on the move almost daily walking great distances in their surveillance of cattle, property, girls, and distant friends. Their exercise seems to be primarily walking, which is done with a brisk, long stride at a rate from 3 to 5 miles per hour. The Masai men rarely participate in maximal effort unless there is a war or other catastrophe. It must be concluded that persistent walking with an expenditure rate of no more than 300 to 500 calories per hour is sufficient to maintain their high degree of fitness.

9. A report of the Food and Nutrition Board, National Academy of Sciences, National Research Council on "Dietary Fat and Human Health." This concludes: Diets very low and conversely, those very high in fat are compatible with low plasma cholesterol concentration. Even diets high in saturated fats are associated with low cholesterol. Undoubtedly other environmental conditions must be taken into account, especially energy expenditure (physical exercise).

IS EXERCISE THE ANSWER?

The foregoing studies would seem to indicate that exercise is a definite factor in blood vessel disease. I do not believe that it is the only factor. Let me give you yet another study which will explain why I feel other elements must be considered. St. Mary's Hospital of London, England did a study of patients on various diets. One group received amounts of corn oil and showed a decrease in serum cholesterol levels. (Does this remind you of the commercials on certain products containing corn oil? These commercials forget to tell you the most important conclusion arrived from this group. Read on.) These patients demonstrated, as a group, more major heart attacks from blood vessel disease than those who took a normal diet! Does this surprise you? What does it mean? The real significance here is the fact that an increase of unsaturated fatty acids in the system increases the need for vitamin E, which acts as an anti-oxidant and prevents the formation of peroxides, a toxic by-product of the metabolism of volatile oils. The possibility that rancid oils, which had been deodorized and clarified, were used is also a factor which

183

we cannot overlook. The use of such oils would have increased even more the need for extra vitamin E. Excessive peroxides in the blood stream cause three major problems:

1. Hemolytic anemia
2. Convulsions
3. Cardiovascular weakness

These three conditions were brought to light in the space program when astronauts were being tested for physical changes due to simulated spaceship environments and developed these symptoms. In trying to determine the cause, a researcher felt that the high oxygen content increased the peroxide formation from unsaturated fatty acids present in the body. Since peroxide formation is normally prevented in the body by an adequate amount of vitamin E present in the blood stream, vitamin E was added to the diets of the astronauts. All symptoms were relieved and all astronauts from then on received extra vitamin E.

And how does this relate to the cholesterol-lowering corn oil diet in which the patients had more coronary artery disease? The toxic peroxides may be the chemical agents which irritated the wall of the blood vessel and produced an emergency situation calling for the blood protein, fibrin, to lay down its 'fish net' threads to protect the artery from leaking. The blood fats, including triglycerides and cholesterol, the minerals in solution including calcium, and other blood ingredients can become involved in the particular area, forming the atheromatous plaque.

The above theory (at this point that is all it is, but a far more defensible one than the present fat intake theory) is further upheld by findings on autopsy that blood vessels are not universally clogged, but only in spotty patches. One researcher has postulated that physical blood vessel abnormalities, causing 'eddy' currents in the blood flow could also explain the lack of total atherosclerosis. The 'eddy currents' would create a particular wear and tear effect causing the lining of the blood vessel wall to either become irritated or wear thin, either of which would cause the laying down of fibrin in an attempt by the body to strengten the area.

Such speculation only further bolsters the theory that some irritation or irritating substance produces changes in the arterial wall which predisposes the atherosclerosis condition. Scientists who work only in the field of blood vessel disease have presented convincing evidence that the atheromateous plaque is only formed after some type of injurious factor changes the cell of the arterial wall from a normal to an abnormal cell. At this time the known injurious factors are:

1. CHEMICAL POISONS — In this category we would have to include the toxins found in cigarette smoking and the heavy concentration of carbon monoxide found in a city street jammed with cars that have their motors running. The mineral cadmium is also highly suspect. Animals given minute amounts of this substance develop atherosclerosis. Where do you get cadmium? From coffee and tea most commonly — five or more cups of either will double your normal intake. The mineral zinc protects against excess cadmium storage in the body, so if you must drink coffee or tea, be sure you supplement with zinc. Another group of chemicals is, interestingly enough, related to cholesterol. When cholesterol is oxidized, certain substances are produced that harm artery walls. The interesting part of this is that the harm usually comes from cholesterol that has been oxidized outside the body (such as charbroiled meat, or deep fat fried foods, or precooked foods) and does not occur with cholesterol that is in the cell. This is another indication that man has set the stage for degenerative disease with his great preoccupation with cooked foods.

2. VIRAL INFECTIONS — These lowly forms of life which multiply at an astronomical rate at just below body temperature can and do create real problems for the individual who does not have a resistance which will withstand their attack. My only comment here is to keep your body as healthy as possible and they don't have a chance.

3. PHYSICAL FACTORS — High blood pressure falls into this category and studies have confirmed the relationship between the incidence of atherosclerosis and high blood pressure. My suggestion here is to read the chapter on "Blood Pressure" for a review of causes and ways to control it and even normalize it. Radiation from x-rays, electronic appliances such as TVs in excess can also set up irritation in the blood vessel wall. Be sure that x-rays are taken only when necessary and don't sit too close to your television.

HOMOGENIZED MILK AS A FACTOR

Another extremely interesting theory has been proposed by Dr. Kurt Oster who feels that the homogenization of milk breaks down the normal-sized fat particles and allows an enzyme called xanthine oxidase to enter the blood stream which, in turn, destroys vital body chemicals that would normally protect the arteries of the heart. To back up his concept, Dr. Oster claims that the death rate from heart disease in different countries is proportionate to how much homogenized milk people drink and also is far less in countries where the people normally boil their milk before drinking — which destroys the xanthine oxidase. I might point out that this same boiling also destroys other good nutrients in the milk, but the point that homogenizing milk releases an enzyme which potentially can injure the blood vessels certainly is in line with the theory presented by other scientists on irritating substances causing cellular changes in the blood vessel wall.

VITAMIN C AS A PROTECTOR

Dr. Constance Spittle, a young English physician, has come up with a study which would indicate that vitamin C may help significantly in preventing the development of atherosclerosis. Through extensive testing, Dr. Spittle found that even on an extremely high cholesterol containing dietary, blood cholesterol levels would actually drop if adequate fresh fruits and vegetables were consumed. This information was then studied and it was determined that vitamin C was possibly the factor responsible for the change. Using this information, she took 25 patients who were known atherosclerotics, and gave them vitamin C. Confusingly, their blood serum cholesterol levels went up! This paradox was resolved when it was determined that this was actually cholesterol which had been literally dissolved from the atheromatous plaque and was now flowing in the blood stream to the liver for use by the body.

A study in Florida had 60 patients with atherosclerosis take large doses of vitamin C — up to 3,000 mg. daily — over an extended period of time. Cholesterol levels did not come down, but no one had a recurrence of heart attack from blood vessel disease and 50 of the 60 showed marked improvement in health. Statistics would tell us that at least 18 of the 60 would have a recurrence of their original problem — heart attack. Dr. Spittle says, "I suggest that atherosclerosis is a long-term deficiency of vitamin C that permits cholesterol levels to build in the arterial system."

I cannot accept that view totally, but am convinced that vitamin C has a protective action in the blood vascular system and probably does work as a transporter of cholesterol to the liver. My objection would lie in the fact that I don't believe that cholesterol, even if super abundant, will just lodge onto a blood vessel. The pumping action of the heart keeps the blood flowing through these vessels and a problem area has to develop before the cholesterol will attach itself to the wall. I personally feel that vitamin C activates an enzyme secreted by the wall of the blood vessel which makes it impossible for cholesterol or other blood fats to accumulate.

WHAT ABOUT THE LOW FAT DIET?

Certain individuals have been given much publicity on a very low fat diet approach to the problem of atherosclerosis. This particular regime also eliminates refined sugar and refined flour. Participants are encouraged to exercise consistently every day. The program seems to work, people with diagnosed atherosclerosis feel better and act better. But I think the emphasis is on the wrong part of the whole program. It is not the low fat factor which is making these people well. It is the elimination of sugar and participation in an exercise program that produces the results. Let me enumerate a few facts:

1. A body which does not receive adequate fat as a part of the diet will become extremely deficient in the fat soluble vitamins A, D, E, and K. Fat is part of the transport mechanism for these vitamins and totally necessary. Eventually all kinds of problems will arise from these deficiencies: premature aging with wrinkling, dry skin appearance, predisposition to infections, particularly of respiratory and urinary tract, sensitivity to light, arthritic symptoms, and perhaps most important — loss of adequate hormone

production leading to sterility and loss of sex drive.

2. The primary fatty acid (stearic acid) that makes up the fat of beef has no effect in raising, but may actually lower serum cholesterol.

3. Skim milk, a product often recommended on these diets, contains appreciable amounts of cholesterol, the very thing they are trying to eliminate.

4. Studies of individuals eating a diet solely made up of eggs, 18 per day, demonstrated a dramatic lowering of serum cholesterol, even though eggs are routinely condemned and ostracized because of a supposed cholesterol increasing effect. Balderdash! (an expletive having the same meaning as 'baloney').

5. The evidence presented at the beginning of this booklet indicated that many very scientific studies proved that the intake of fat had nothing to do with blood vessel disease. Exercise was the most common factor in preventing heart attacks from blood vessel disease.

SO YOU MEAN TO SAY THAT DIET HAS NOTHING TO DO WITH ATHEROSCLEROSIS?

I definitely do not mean to give the impression that diet has nothing to do with blood vessel disease. I have cited the studies on vitamin E and vitamin C and their relationship to prevention. I highly endorse a high protein, high fiber, medium fat, low carbohydrate diet as a means of creating the most disease resistant body possible. The Creative Restoration Diet printed at the end of this book becomes an easy to follow, common-sense approach to eating with plenty of variety. Do consider following such an eating plan whether you have or do not have atherosclerosis.

On the other hand, certain evidence would make me reach the conclusion that a high unsaturated fat diet could be harmful as could a very low fat diet. Experience will tell most of us that moderation is the best path to travel in a search for health.

SYNOPSIS

1. The eating of cholesterol containing foods does not raise cholesterol or the incidence of atherosclerosis.
2. Butter is a far better food, containing vitamin E and other food factors, than its touted replacement margarine. Actually, most margarines are more saturated than butter (even though advertisements would falsely lead you to believe differently).
3. Eggs are one of the finest foods that man can eat. Their consumption will not affect your cholesterol or blood vessel disease incidence except to lower your cholesterol and make your body more disease resistant.
4. Try to engage in physical exercise each and every day to avoid atherosclerosis.
5. Supplement your diet with vitamins C and E and the mineral zinc for further protection.
6. Use a high protein, high fiber, medium fat, low carbohydrate diet as the outline of your eating habits.
7. Do not drink homogenized milk, use raw or just the cream.

HOW ABOUT CHELATION?

Many have heard in recent years of a miraculous method of reducing atherosclerosis by the injection of a synthetic amino acid (EDTA) into the blood stream. Although it has no specific action on the cholesterol or triglycerides in the atheromatous plaque, it disrupts the plaque by picking up the minerals contained therein and eliminating them via the kidneys. The effects are dramatic in a short period of time, I have seen individuals with advanced senility because of decreased blood supply to the brain recover within three weeks. Others who could not walk across a room without taking nitroglycerin for the angina pains, were out playing golf within six weeks.

Such incredible results can lead to complacency, but beware! This is strictly emergency procedure in my opinion, and does nothing to correct the cause for the problem existing in the first place. A person who has been chelated and who continues to ignore the basic principles of good health maintenance will be right back in the doctor's office within two years for more chelation.

Preventive chelation can be accomplished by the oral ingestion of amino acid chelated minerals in a formulation designed to be compatible with the blood chemistry. Here is a suggested formula:

Calcium (amino acid chelate) 375mg
Magnesium (amino acid chelate) 180mg
Phosphorus (amino acid complex) 75mg
Iodine (kelp) .... .225mg
Iron (amino acid chelate) 15mg
Copper (amino acid chelate) 3mg
Zinc (amino acid chelate) 15mg
Chromium (amino acid chelate) 1.5mg
Potassium (amino acid complex) 99mg
Manganese (amino acid chelate) 30mg
Selenium (yeast) 5mcg

Chapter 13

HEART ATTACK

HEART PAIN
(YOUR ANGINA PECTORIS)

DEFINITION

Angina pectoris is a name given to a specific type of pain which usually occurs in the left chest in front of the heart sometimes extending into the left arm or neck. It is a temporary type of pain, meaning that it will subside soon without any sort of treatment aside from rest. It develops into acute myocardial ischemia, meaning lack of blood to heart muscle, or coronary heart disease when the pain persists beyond the temporary point. In reality, the pain occurs when there is a shortage of oxygen being delivered to the heart muscle or part thereof in a given period of time. The pain disappears when the oxygen supply is improved. Thus, reducing the work level of the heart by rest may relatively increase the available oxygen supply sufficiently to alleviate the angina pectoris. Obviously, then, when angina develops, one should rest.

CARDIOVASCULAR SYSTEM

Only a brief summary of the cardiovascular system is presented here. This system consists of the heart and two systems of arteries and veins interconnected by capillary networks. The first or systemic circulation is the one that supplies the whole body with oxygenated blood while the second or pulmonic circulation is the one that takes used blood to the lungs to be oxygenated. The cardiovascular system is called a closed system, meaning that it is circular in nature, hence the same blood is used over and over again, being cleansed in certain areas and saturated with nutrients in other areas so that it can carry on its functions of feeding and removing waste products from the tissues. In the systemic circulation the arterial blood is oxygenated or carries a full load of oxygen while the veins carry used or deoxygenated blood back to the heart. The blood then passes into the pulmonary circulation where the arteries carry used blood to the lungs to be oxygenated and the veins carry oxygenated blood back to the heart to be sent into the systemic circulation to give oxygen to the tissues. Round and round it goes; equivalent to 4,300 gallons per day with over 100,000 heart contractions in a 24 hour period.

THE HEART

The anatomical structure of the heart includes three separate layers of heart tissue. The endocardium or lining of the heart chambers, the myocardium or muscular component which is the contracting part of the heart, and the epicardium or pericardium which carries the nerves and arteries to the heart muscle itself and is protective from outside influences. Please note that the heart muscle is not supplied its own oxygen need from the blood which passes through the chambers of the heart, but by special arteries (called coronary arteries), which pass via the outer heart layer into the heart muscle.

There are four heart chambers in the heart, two on the right and two on the left. The left side is concerned with the systemic circulation while the right is a part of the pulmonic circulation. The chambers are separated by valves which prevent backflow of blood into the wrong chamber. Each chamber has a valve at its exit point. The mouths of the coronary arteries are located just outside the aortic valve in the aorta which is the main artery of the systemic circulation.

Filling the coronary arteries with blood is a definite mechanical problem for two reasons. One is that when the aortic valves are open, they block the free flow of blood into the coronaries. The second is, when the heart muscle is pumping blood, much pressure is created within the muscle itself which actually prevents blood flow in the coronaries.

Therefore, blood must flow into the heart muscle when it is relaxed, i.e. between pulse beats. At this stage, the aortic valves are closed to allow free flow of blood into the coronary arteries and the blood pressure within the aorta is at a maximum again aiding coronary blood flow.

MECHANISM FOR REDUCED BLOOD FLOW INTO THE CORONARIES

Any factor which reduces coronary blood flow actually reduces the oxygen supply going to the heart muscle and potentially reduces this flow sufficiently to cause angina pectoris. As noted before, the coronary flow is reduced to nothing while the heart is contracting. This is normal. But after the contraction, there should be a rest period for the heart, which allows the coronaries to fill with blood. A

195

number of problems may occur because of various factors which may cause a muscle spasm or "charley horse" of the heart. The coronary flow is maximal when the aortic valves close. Therefore, when there is aortic valve incompetency or failure to close securely, the coronary flow is jeopardized since aortic blood pressure falls to low levels when it should be high. This becomes very serious and imcompatible with life when the valve is totaly incompetent. When the heart rate is too rapid due to stress or exertion, the muscle contraction time occupies too much of the contraction cycle time. After all, there must be enough time for the coronaries to become filled with blood to unload its supply of oxygen. Finally, there may be some sort of mechanical blockage of the blood flow in the heart caused by hardened arteries, embolus (foreign body) or such. An infarct is the point of blockage and may result from local problems like hardened arteries or from a remote area like a blood clot or embolus floating in the blood stream that becomes lodged in a coronary artery. Each infarct causes an area of ischemia or lack of blood supply in the heart muscle serviced by that particular coronary artery.

ABNORMALITIES THAT CAUSE
REDUCED CORONARY BLOOD FLOW

The above reasons for reduced blood flow in the coronaries can be caused individually or collectively by the following:

1. Stress causes increased reactions in the body and thus makes demands on the cardiovascular system for more oxygen laden blood supply to the glands and all cells. This is like emotional experiences which make the muscles of the body tense and the mind race. Both cause need for more oxygen, hence more blood flow.

2. Anemia reduces the oxygen carrying capability of the blood. Therefore, more blood volume per unit of time is needed to supply basic oxygen needs to the tissues.

3. Smoking creates more work for the liver to detoxify the toxic products found in cigarette smoke. When the liver works harder, it needs more oxygen and hence more blood supply.

4. The flu is a toxic situation where body defenses are being taxed heavily, thus demanding more oxygen from the circulation. This latter picture is complicated by congestion in the lungs so the oxygenation of the blood is less efficient thus even more blood is needed to supply the extra amount needed to enhance the defensive reactions of the body.

5. An enlarged heart demands more blood supply. It works like this: if the valve(s) are incompetent or fail to close securely, some of the blood flows backwards with each beat. When backflow happens, the heart chamber behind the valve gradually becomes dilated due to the extra amount of blood contained in the chamber. As this stretching or dilation increases, the heart muscle increases in size, called hypertrophy, to compensate for the extra load, just like your arm muscles increase in size when you hammer more nails. One peculiarity here is that it is the size of the individual muscle cells that enlarge and not the formation of more muscle cells. Likewise, there is not an increase in the number of coronary arteries to supply extra blood to the larger cells. Naturally, there is a limit as to how much circulation the coronaries can provide so when the muscle enlargement increases to the point of exceeding its available blood supply, angina pectoris develops and becomes a chronic way of life. Then we have frequent, prolonged episodes of angina pectoris which are caused by relatively minor degrees of physical activity.

6. Additionally, but not least by any means, sugar and processed carbohydrates. Here we see that sugar and

processed carbohydrates demand B complex vitamins in order to be processed through the metabolic biochemical channels within the body. When the B vitamins (B vitamins have been removed by processing sugar cane and sugar beets to produce pure white sugar, etc.) are stolen from other areas of metabolism or biochemical activity in the body creating deficiencies in these metabolic areas, problems can result in these remote areas. One such metabolic area or physiologic system affected is the nervous system. In relation to the heart this means that nerve control of the rate and rhythm of the heart can be altered and the development of cardiac arrythmias, or abnormal pulsations like tachycardia, auricular fibrillation, atrial flutter, ventricular fibrillation and flutter occur. These arrhythmias can rapidly become disabling and even life and death situations. In the process, the arrhythmias are quite capable of causing gross reduction in coronary blood flow, hence angina pectoris.

7. Synthetic fats and chemicals in the diet and environment are taken into the body one way or another. These substances are not foods since they do not contain the naturally associated synergistic micronutrients. Therefore, they must steal the essential vitamins, minerals, enzymes, etc., from other areas of metabolism in order to be metabolized out of the body. Naturally, we then find various nutritional deficiencies like vitamin B complex, E, and others as well as minerals. Enzymes and even sub-atomic substances are lacking in this picture as well.

8. Obviously, hardened arteries cause a reduction in blood flow per unit of time. When coupled with any of the above mentioned factors, the probability of development of angina pectoris increases. Hardened arteries and arteriolar spasm are prime considerations in any angina pectoris problems.

PREVENTIVE MEASURES

The name of the game is that a healthy cell is not a sick cell. Sick cells need an extra supply of all the various nutrients, known and unknown, to nourish the body, including oxygen. A good diet should contain an abundance and variety of fresh, raw foods. The more the better. Such foods should include vegetables and fruits as well as lipids (fats) and proteins. For example, many large salads should be the password of the day. Raw milk and raw fertile eggs are a good source of lipids and proteins. Meat may be eaten as desired except for the processed meats like bacon and ham, sausage and bologna, etc., which should be avoided. One should also arrange to avoid chemicalized or hormonized meats.

B COMPLEX

More specifically, for angina pectoris and for the prevention of an aggravation of such, one should consume an abundance of the "particularly friendly toward the heart" nutrients. Among these important supplements we find B complex. B complex is a must for 'heart-nerve' integrity. When suffering from angina, one should always be very careful to 'balance' the vitamin B group. As an example if B-1 or thiamine is used without an adequate amount of B-2 or riboflavin, the problem of angina may actually be aggrevated rather than helped. This occurs because of the constricting effect that B-1 exerts on the coronary vessels in B-2 deficient states.

VITAMIN E

Vitamin E is another important factor in guarding against

angina pectoris. The action of vitamin E is to enhance the utilization of oxygen by the tissues. It also increases the blood supply in the coronary arteries and arterioles, hence tending to improve coronary circulation.

CALCIUM

Calcium is important in reducing irritability of the nerves and muscles so that the possibility of "Charley Horses" is decreased. Other factors necessary for calcium utilization include the proper balance of sodium, magnesium, phosphorus, potassium, as well as vitamin D. Proper pH of the stomach with adequate hydrochloric acid is also necessary. They all work together to metabolize calcium.

POTASSIUM

Potassium is very important unto itself. It is the intracellular electrolyte of great importance as is sodium for the extracellular fluid. Lack of potassium causes a weakness of the nerves supplying the heart muscle. Failure of the heart muscle means that the heart is no longer capable of sending enough blood out into the peripheral circulation to nourish the cells.

SAMPLE FORMULA OF A BALANCED
VITAMIN-MINERAL COMPLEX

Vitamin A	25,000IU	Folic Acid	400mcg
Vitamin D	400IU	Biotin	100mcg
Vitamin E	400IU	Calcium	1,000mg
Vitamin C	1,200mg	Magnesium	400mg
Vitamin B-1	60mg	Phosphorus	150mg
Vitamin B-2	60mg	Potassium	99mg
Vitamin B-6	60mg	Iron	15mg
Vitamin B-12	100mcg	Iodine	225mcg

Niacin	30mg	Copper	2mg
Niacinamide	30mg	Chromium	200mcg
Pantothenic Acid	100mg	Manganese	15 mg
PABA	60 mg	Selenium	100mcg
Choline	60mg	Zinc	15mg
Inositol	60mg		

HOW ABOUT CHELATION

Many have heard in recent years of a miraculous method of reducing atherosclerosis or hardened arteries by the injection of a synthetic amino acid (EDTA) into the blood stream. Although it has no specific action on cholesterol or triglycerides in the atheromatous plaque, it disrupts the plaque by picking up the minerals contained therein and eliminating them via the kidneys. The effects may be dramatic in a short period of time. Some who could not walk across a room without taking nitroglycerin for the angina pains, were out playing golf within six weeks or so.

To me, EDTA chelation technique is capable of reversing certain hardened artery development but does not correct the basic cause. It is not and should not be considered a preventive technique in the same sense as nutritional techniques are truly preventive.

Preventive chelation can be accomplished by the oral ingestion of amino acid chelated minerals in a formulation designed to be compatible with the blood chemistry. Here is a suggested formula:

Calcium (amino acid chelate) 375mg
Magnesium (amino acid chelate) 180mg
Phosphorus (amino acid complex) 75mg
Iodine (kelp) .... .225mg
Iron (amino acid chelate) 15mg
Copper (amino acid chelate) 3mg
Zinc (amino acid chelate) 15mg
Chromium (amino acid chelate) 200mcg

Potassium (amino acid complex) 99mg
Manganese (amino acid chelate) 30mg
Selenium (yeast) 15mcg

ENZYME THERAPY

Enzymes are the chemical backbone of metabolism. Nothing happens in the metabolic or internal biochemical area without enzymes. Chemical reactions that could take 100 years to happen in a test tube can be made to occur instantaneously in the body by the action of enzymes. Therefore, an abundance of enzymes in the system can be beneficial in times of stress and peril. This abundance of enzymes can be accomplished by oral administration of enzyme preparations.

Actually, there are two distinctive areas of enzyme activity within the system. One is in the digestive tract where enzymes play an integral part in the digestion of foods, into utilizable nutrients. The other is internal or within the cellular structures. All biochemical or metabolic reactions need enzymes for activation. Both enzyme systems are strengthened by the consumption of enzyme laden foods. Since heat destroys enzymes, this means raw foods.

ENZYME FORMULA

Betaine 60mg
Pancreatin 4x 75mg
Pepsin 1:3000 .... 35mg
Papain 50mg
Lipase 50mg
Ext. Ox Bile 65mg
Rennin 15mg
Glutamic Acid Hydrochloride 10mg

HORMONES

Hormone balance is a must for good health. On occasion, some gross abnormalities in the coronaries can be found when lack of the thyroid hormone, thyroxin, exists. When there is lack of this hormone, hypothyroidism is present wherein there tends to be more hardened arteries than when normal thyroid functions exist. Obviously, angina pectoris by itself is a major stress, so the adrenals (anti-stress glands) should be supported and strengthened. This means more vitamin C and pantothenic acid intake. It also means raw adrenocortical tissue supplementation (DNA support). In fact, one suspects that there is a generalized hypoglandular situation in existence when angina pectoris is present. In general, polyglandular systemic support, i.e., a balanced multi-glandular approach, is indicated rather than single entity therapy.

FEMALE

Ovarian Substance	60mg
Whole Pituitary Substance	20mg
Adrenal Substance	60mg
Thymus Substance	60mg
Pancreas Substance	60mg
Kidney Substance	60mg
Heart Substance	60mg
Ribonucleic Acid (RNA)	60mg

MALE

Prostate Substance	60mg
Whole Pituitary Substance	20mg
Adrenal Substance	60mg
Thymus Substance	60mg
Pancreas Substance	60mg
Kidney Substance	60mg
Heart Substance	60mg
Ribonucleic Acid (RNA)	60mg

EXERCISE AND REST

Two other very important factors must be considered — exercise and rest. It is very true that exercise will increase the circulation, thus the oxygenation of the tissues is improved and more waste products are removed from the cellular area. This is a beneficial factor and should be encouraged but a word of caution is to be considered. Exercise can be overdone and cause more problems rather than instigating improvement.

Thus, all exercise suggestions are purely relevant to the individual patient. In general, one wishes to do as much as possible without causing an aggravation. Even if the patient is only able to move the big toes, that is to be done routinely every day. If he is able to walk, that is to be done. Exercise, to be effective must challenge the cardiovascular system to do a little better each day, not necessarily a lot better. Increase the exercise modules slowly so that one does not create an emergency cardiovascular situation. Stay within the capability of the heart as it exists. You cannot pull yourself up by bootstraps. It must be a building process wherein the heart is gradually urged to do better as it is being freely supplied with all basic nutrients.

Rest, the other side of the coin to exercise, is also important. Even though one does exercise, he needs rest too. For invalids, eight or nine or more hours at night and some time in bed morning and afternoon is needed. Maybe more sitting in an easy chair is indicated as well. All of this is subject to individual evaluation. Point to remember, one can cause irreparable heart damage by over-exercise and under-rest programs at the wrong time. Timing is important.

THE CORONARY BYPASS PROCEDURE

The coronary bypass procedure is amazingly popular

today. It is anticipated that some 6,000 such operations will be performed this year throughout the country. The procedure is to transplant a small section of vein from a remote area like the leg into the coronary artery circuit. The coronary artery between the heart and infarct area is opened and the transplant is attached. The vein graft is then looped over the infarct and attached to a good section of the artery on the other side of the infarct. With the fabulous surgical techniques used these days, this operation carries a relatively low mortality rate as compared to non-surgical methods now in use.

However, this technique does not do anything about correcting the cause of the infarct. In fact, it is generally known that the transplanted vein develops hardening comparable to the original situation within a period of about two years. Net gain for the patient is about two years of relatively comfortable life. Contrarily, change in life style is necessary for correction of cause and thus becomes a permanent healing.

SYNOPSIS

If you wish to overcome angina pectoris, the following program is a must:

1. Stop smoking.
2. Don't drink coffee, tea, alcohol, cola drinks, or high sugar beverages.
3. Be sure your intake of calcium is adequate.
4. Don't use common table salt. Substitute herbs or a combination potassium-sodium salt.
5. Do drink lots of pure water — about 2 quarts daily.
6. Use the Liver-Kidney Cleansing Diet.

7. Follow the cleansing by adhering to the Ceative Restoration Diet as your food guidelines.
8. If you have hypertension complicated with arteriosclerosis or atherosclerosis, it might be worth your while to consider chelation therapy from a physician to cleanse your arteries.
9. To support all body functions, their restoration to normal and the maintenance of the functions, use a broad spectrum vitamin and mineral supplement program.
10. Apply the principles of botanical medicine by using herbs to assist in cleansing the liver. Purified garlic is a good systemic stimulant.

In order to accomplish desirable heart status, one must be willing to change his life style. Obviously, since trouble now exists in your body, a change in life style will be necessary to effect improvement.

Chapter 14

FIRMING UP EXERCISES

Much has been written and promised in spas and other places that certain exercises will help you lose weight. With the proper nutritional program as an assistant, this can be very true. I hope in this chapter to offer you particular exercises which will help you to firm up the 'sags and bags' that can be the result of a concentrated weight reduction program.

I might point out at this time that the physically fit person is able to withstand fatigue for longer periods than the unfit, is better able to tolerate physical and mental stress, has a stronger and more efficient heart, and usually is more mentally alert. Also, for those of you with back pain, the most common cause of this malady is weak back muscles.

The major purpose of weight control is to reduce the amount of fat on the body and to increase the amount of muscle. It is in reality a program of fat control rather than weight control. This control can be exerted only by coupling a sensible dietary program with a regular balanced program of exercise.

When we eat, the food is absorbed and then either used up for energy or stored as fat. The more we consume, and the less we use, the more can be stored in the body in the form of fat. The human body is not like a car's gas tank that will overflow when full. Our bodies accept all the calories that we put into them, and store those which we do not use. It is extremely logical that an increase of daily exercise will use up more energy than normal and we will not store as much.

The dietary program outlined at the back of this booklet has been proven successful by many people. It combines a good negative calorie program with a high protein intake necessary to build up muscle tissue used in exercise. My opinion on fasting for weight loss is considerably weighted by knowledge that most individuals who use this technique have a rebound weight gain as soon as they come off the fast. On the other hand, an educated diet and exercise plan can be something you can follow all the time for increased energy and enthusiasm.

GENERAL EXERCISE

There are many forms of general exercise, but the one which excels all others both in ability and convenience as well as results, is walking. The only requirements are that you walk with a definite purpose in mind and spend at least 45 minutes a day walking. You cannot amble along as if you are walking a toy poodle, instead you must stride out at a pace about equivalent to three miles per hour. In your car, that seems like standing still, but try walking next to a car going that fast to get the feel of it. Other tips are to park your car at least a block away from your shopping door and walk; if you use public transportation, try getting off a few blocks from your destination and walking the balance of the way. Use stairways instead of elevators or escalators. Probably the most difficult lesson most individuals have to learn is that exercise really creates energy by converting fat into energy. (See the chapter on OVERWEIGHT for more detailed information.)

When we speak of an overall exercise program we should never forget swimming. Although the weather will restrict this on certain days of the year, many physical fitness educators consider swimming as the finest full body exercise. Again, we have to emphasize the duration and vigor with which you swim. You can't do five laps in the pool and spend the next hour sunning yourself and consider that as exercise.

There are many other forms of exercise which often are a unilateral type of motion such as tennis or golf — although both of these exercise the entire body quite equally except one arm. Golf also offers excellent walking opportunity combined with sport, so forget the cart.

Isometric exercises were all the rage a few years ago and then seem to have died down in popularity. They are still effective means of exercising when the circumstances do not permit you to do your regular routine. Simple ones include:

1. Tone up your shoulder and arm muscles and bust while sitting at a desk. Place hands on desk, palms down, elbows bent, and press down trying to lift body from chair. Hold the pressure for about 10 seconds. Relax and repeat.
2. Firm up that belly. While waiting for a red light to turn, contract abdominal muscles and hold for about 10 seconds. Relax and repeat.
3. Help for your double chin. This should probably be done in private, because others who might observe you will be sure you are in terrible agony. Make a horrible grimace with your facial muscles, taking particular care to put the neck and under chin muscles into the act. Hold for about 10 seconds. Relax and try another.

4. Trim up the calf of your leg. Sit upright in a chair and push your feet against the floor as if you were trying to push right on through. Hold for about 10 seconds and relax. Repeat several times during the day.

SPECIFIC EXERCISES

As we lose weight, there often is a problem with certain areas where the fat has melted and the skin did not tighten up immediately or the muscle tone was so poor that characteristic 'pouching' occurs which is ugly to say the least. The following exercises are designed to assist you in firming up the muscles to give a pleasing contour to the body again.

They should be practiced religiously at least once a day and twice a day if time permits. There is no better way to start the day than with an exercise program, it gets the circulation going and things just seem to go easier afterward. Conversely, there is no better way to relieve tensions at the end of the day than a good round of controlled exercise. For most, it works better than Sominex ever dreamed of. It also is fun to see yourself progressing to more vigorous exercise and reap the benefits from improved health.

Although the model for the exercises is a woman, these exercises work just as well for the male as they do the female. Any of the arm exercises help develop the pectoral muscles which assist in firming and expanding the chest in the male and assist in providing an uplift to the bust in the female. There are, of course, hundreds of exercises which can be used, far more than can be put in this small booklet. The ones I have chosen excel in what they are intended to accomplish — you can easily see how they can be expanded or varied for your own personal needs.

You will note that the model is using a slant board to do these exercises. Although a slant board is not absolutely necessary, it certainly makes it more convenient, and is more comfortable than the floor even if carpeted.

FIRM UP THE BUTTOCKS AND THIGHS

1. Assume a basic hand and knee position. Try to keep back straight.
2. Bring left knee up toward chest.
3. Extend leg backward to a level plane with your buttock.
4. Bring knee back up to knee-chest position without touching floor.
5. Extend leg backward to a level plane with your buttock.

This is repeated 10 times with the left leg and then 10 times with the right leg. After you no longer tire you can increase up to 20 or 25 repeats. This exercise can take that sagging rump and firm it up to the pleasing contours of the 20s.

FIRM UP THE BUTTOCKS AND THIGHS

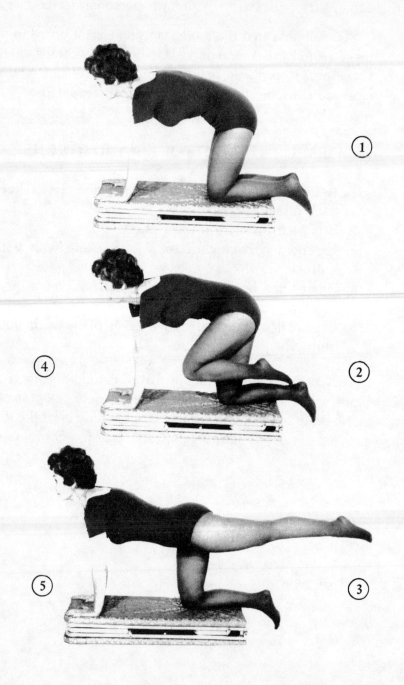

EXERCISE FOR A FLAT TUMMY

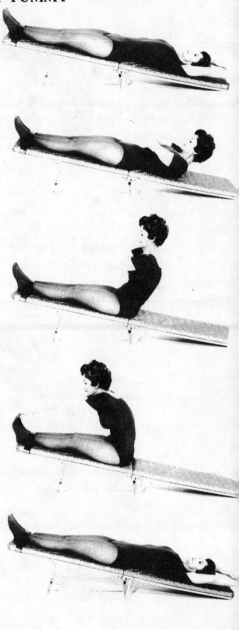

1. Lie on slantboard with arms overhead, palms up.

2. Reach forward with arms, arching back.

3. Continue reaching for your toes, keeping firm control.

4. Touch toes, making sure knees do not bend.

5. Return slowly to reclining position.

Repeat exercise five times to begin with and slowly increase as your muscle tone allows.

EXERCISE FOR THE JOWLS AND CHIN

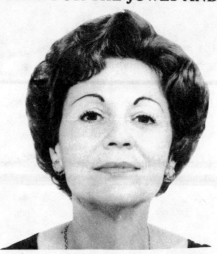

This exercise is difficult to explain, but easy to do. Look straight ahead and put a half smile on your face with the chin pointing outward.

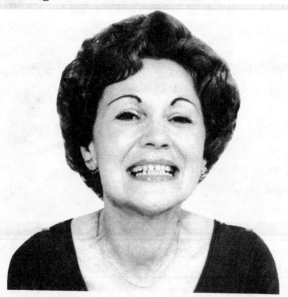

Now spread the lower jaw sideways using the muscles along both sides of the jaw and under the chin and jaws. It might help to say a-a-a-a-r-r-gh in a very disgusted manner. You should feel all the flesh under the jaw and chin draw up very tight. Hold for count of five, repeat 10 times.

214

ERASE THE FLAB ON YOUR ARMS

1. Lie on floor with legs elevated. Arms are on the floor, close to your body. Backs of hands rest on the floor,
2. Slowly bring hands into an upright position, with palms facing toward you until in a straight up attitude.

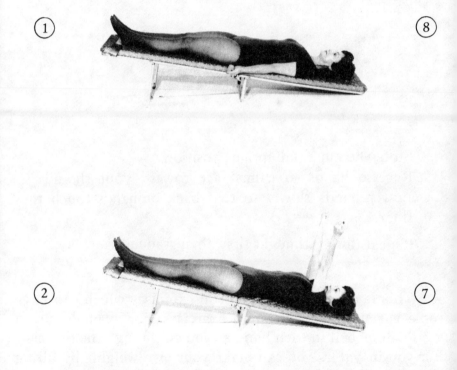

3. Turn hands so palms face your feet.
4. Slowly lower arms back over your head to the floor, un til backs of hands rest on floor.
5. Slowly raise arms.

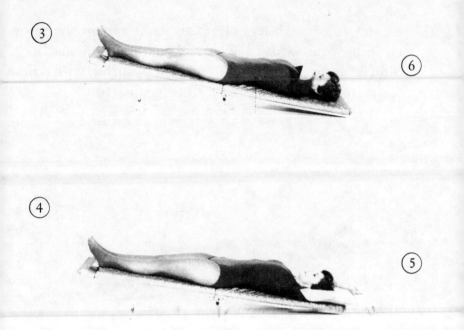

6.   Stop when in a full upright position.
7.   Reverse hands so palms face toward your shoulders.
8.   Lower hands slowly so that back of hands touch the floor.

Repeat this 10 times at first, then gradually increase.

This is one of those delightful exercises which can have some variations for advanced exercises. For example: use a 2-5 lb. dumbbell in each hand as you go through the exercise. For you inovators you can make your own weights by filling a cloth bag with salt to the desired weight (be sure the bag is sealed well).

216

SLIM UP KNEES, CALVES, AND ANKLES

A fabulous exercise for the leg, particularly for the knee, calf and ankle. It is simple to do and will trim those areas in a hurry if you do the exercise every day.

1. Lie on your back, arms extended at shoulder level. Have your palms up, knees bent. Feet should be flat, close to hips.

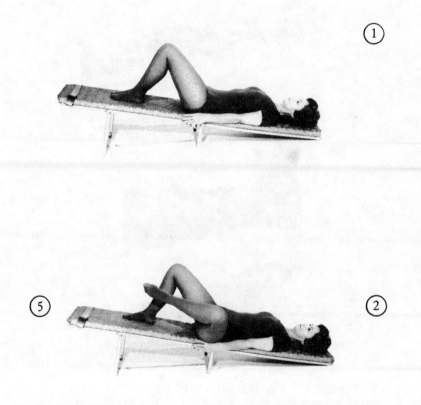

2. Slowly raise the left leg, keeping it bent and turn the knee out as if you were going to lie it flat.

217

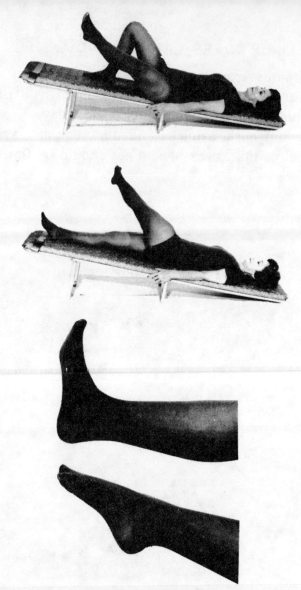

3. Now straighten the leg out, and . . .
4. Cross the leg over the other, pointing across the room.
5. Flex the foot - then point the toes - repeat 5 times.
6. Bend the leg back and place foot in original position.
7. Do this exercise 10 times. Then change legs and do the exercise with the other leg 10 times. Increase as you get stronger.

Exercise for Firming all Muscles
in Legs, Thighs and Tummy
(It also loosens up your back)

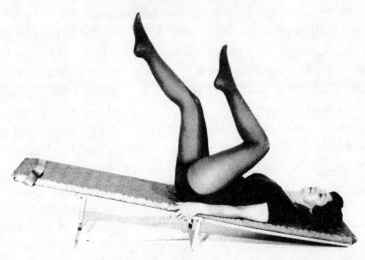

1. Lying on slant board, raise both legs and bicycle. Do for 15 seconds then:

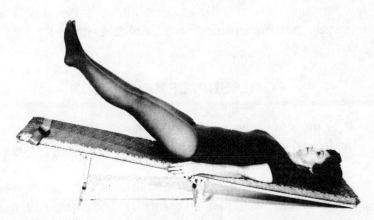

2. Bring legs together about 18″ above slantboard and hold for count of three. Lower 6 inches and hold for count of 3. Lower 6 inches and hold for count of 3 again and then lower to board. Repeat entire exercise bicycling and leg holds 5 times. Increase as muscles tone and firm up.

NUTRITIONAL PROGRAM

Serious weight loss programs require serious attention to detail. If you want best results, follow the program very precisely and the results will amaze even you. It is true that the first few pounds come off easier than those that follow, since the excess fluid which was trapped within your cells with toxic waste products is eliminated. Then the conversion of fat to glycogen to glucose is set into effect and you continue to lose weight in an orderly fashion. You can expect to lose from 4 to 7 pounds the first week and from ¼ to ½ pound daily thereafter. At times your weight will seem to plateau for a day or so, but this is normal and will not be a stopping point. Just continue the program and the weight losing process will take over again.

There are a variety of very good weight reduction programs on the market today — with most of them using the principle of high protein intakes as their basis. There are slight variations as to adjunctive products to enhance a particular program, so I will discuss such variations that I am familiar with. If I leave one out, it is because I am unaware, not necessarily because it is no good.

FOOD SUPPLEMENTATION

It is my contention that everyone needs a good multi-vitamin and mineral supplement today — whether they are on a weight losing regime or not. The foods which we purchase are often grown on soils which have been depleted from essential elements and growth has been forced with the use of chemical fertilizers. We are under great stress today in our society, requiring more B-complex vitamins; subjected to smog which raises our need for vitamin E, government studies indicate almost 50% of our diets are calcium deficient, 30% are vitamin A deficient, iron deficiency anemia is rampant in our women, and on and on. Many of the vitamins and minerals enter into the complex metabolic process in which we convert the food we eat into energy and new cells.

SPECIALTY ADDITIONS

The Kelp-Lecithin B-6 formula has had a rebirth in many programs. This was a proven reducing aid which had a large group of devotees in the not too distant past. The kelp does synergize thyroid function for some, the lecithin does help to emulsify fat, and the vitamin B-6 helps in protein metabolism and in getting rid of excess fluids as well as entering into the fat conversion process. So, all in all, such a formula could enhance the basic high protein approach.

Then we have those who add betaine hydrochloride and/or pepsin to their particular program because, on a high protein diet, the secret is in the digestion and assimilation. Hydrochloric acid and pepsin are absolutely essential for this process to be properly carried out. It might also interest you to know that approximately 50% of the people over 40 years of age have low level or insufficient hydrochloric acid. Again — a good product as an adjunct.

Fiber, in one form or another is also often recommended because the high protein diet can be low in adequate fiber which may tend to constipation. Some will recommend the fiber be put in the protein shake, others use a tablet form — the important thing is to get adequate elimination and a shorter digestive tract time, which the fiber definitely accomplishes. I do endorse this approach because of the many, many benefits to general health it also effects.

Another factor is the concommitant use of herbs. I know of reducing programs which rely heavily on herbs to quench the appetite — and they have good results. If such an assist is what it takes to get the weight off, then by all means use it.

BASIC HIGH PROTEIN PROGRAM

Before we lay out the program, let us discuss the possible problems which might come up by following it.

1. Constipation — increase fiber in diet, using plenty of water with the fiber. It may be millers bran, a bran type tablet, psyllium seed powder, raw cabbage (about a cup to a cup and a half daily), or any of a number of other high fiber foods.
2. Excessive hunger — this is not often experienced, since the diet is so high in protein which provides high levels of energy, but if it should become a problem, just take another protein shake when you get hungry — you might even try adding a raw egg to this one.
3. Nausea, Headaches — it has often been reported that this program actually has alleviated headaches and stomach upset because it tends to normalize the body chemistry, but in some individuals, there may be a sudden release of toxins which will make you feel temporarily lousy. Under such circumstances, the best approach is to flood the body with liquids — water in particular and make sure the bowels are open. It will clear up rapidly.

RULES:

1. You must make two meals per day of the protein shake. It does not help, in fact it hinders your progress, if you miss one of these.

2. Use the supplements as directed. Some of them are very important to synergize the changes in metabolism which must take place.
3. You must get some form of fat in your diet daily — the use of full fat milk, or the addition of oil to the shake are the easiest way to achieve the intake. Fats are necessary for the formation of hormones without which body processes stop.
4. Exercise faithfully every day — walking, tennis, golf, swimming, isometrics/calisthenics, try taking your spouse out to a dance and dance every dance for a couple of hours, instead of being a spectator.

REGIME

TWO MEALS PER DAY: PROTEIN SHAKE
    2 Tablespoonsful Protein Powder
    8 oz. full fat milk
    3 ice cubes
    (Optional)
    2 strawberries . . . or
    ¼ banana . . . or
    2 tablespoonsful cantaloupe . . . or
    1 egg
    Vanilla, lemon, butterscotch, etc. flavoring
    ½ teaspoon honey if needed

MAJOR MEAL: Many feel if this meal is consumed at lunchtime, the weight loss will be enhanced. It is rather difficult for everyone to abide by this, and such exceptional results have been achieved by making this the evening meal that it is really a personal choice.

- Large serving of protein food such as meat, fish, chicken, turkey, cheese, nutmeats, seeds. At least two cups of raw greens, including cabbage, celery, bell pepper, cauliflower, spinach, lettuce, alfalfa and bean sprouts, green beans, parsley, jicama, etc. You may use a vinegar and oil dressing if you wish. You may use a cooked vegetable from the 3% list at the end of this chapter.

After your goal has been reached, you may choose judiciously from the 3% and 6% vegetables and fruits to maintain your weight. Remember that somehow you must burn up that energy you derive from food, so exercise is an all important factor in the overall plan.

CLASSIFICATION OF FOODS
(According to Carbohydrate Content)

VEGETABLES

3 PERCENT	6 PERCENT	15 PERCENT	20 PERCENT	25 PERCENT
Asparagus	Beans, string	Artichokes	Beans, dired	Rice, boiled
Bean sprouts	Beets	Beans, kidney	Beans, lima	Potato, sweet
Beet greens	Brussel sprouts	Hominy	Corn	Yams
Broccoli	Carrots	Oyster plant	Potato, white	
Cabbage	Chives	Parsnips		
Cauliflower	Collards	Peas, green		
Celery	Dandelion			
Chard, swiss	greens			
Cucumber	Eggplant			
Endive	Kale			
Lettuce	Kohlrabi			
Mushrooms	Leeks			
Mustard	Okra			
greens	Onions			
Radishes	Parsley			
Sauerkraut	Peppers, red			
Spinach	Pimento			
Squash	Pumpkin			
Tomatoes	Rutabagas			
Tomato Juice	Turnips			
Turnip greens				
Water Cress				

FRUITS

3 PERCENT	6 PERCENT	15 PERCENT	20 PERCENT	25 PERCENT
Cantaloupe	Apricots	Apples	Bananas	
Rhubarb	Blackberries	Blueberries	Figs	
Strawberries	Cranberries	Cherries	Prunes	
Watermelon	Currants	Grapes		
	Gooseberries	Kumquats		
	Grapefruit	Loganberries		
	Guava	Mangoes		
	Melons	Mulberries		
	Lemons	Pears		
	Limes	Pineapple		
	Oranges	Pomegranates		
	Papayas			
	Peaches			
	Plums			
	Raspberries			
	Tangerines			

Chapter 15

YOUR BLOOD PRESSURE

It is obvious that an in-depth study of the circulatory system is not possible in this chapter. However, by the time you have completed the reading of this, you will have a basic understanding of your internal plumbing, why so many people have problems with it and, even more important, how you can reduce your chances of developing problems or overcome the ones you have existing in your blood vessel system.

THE HEART

At the center of the entire cardio-vascular (heart-blood vessel) system is the heart. It is a muscular organ with four chambers sealed off from each other by valves which work to control the blood flow throughout the internal areas of the heart. The blood which comes back to the heart is loaded with carbon dioxide and is routed to the lungs for an exchange of the carbon dioxide with oxygen which is so essential for life. The oxygen-rich blood then goes back to the heart and is pumped out into the general circulation. The following diagram represents the flow of blood which travels an incredible 60,000 miles through a variety of large and very small blood vessels. The heart pumps the equivalent of 4,300 gallons of fluid in any given day with over 100,000 contractions in a 24-hour period.

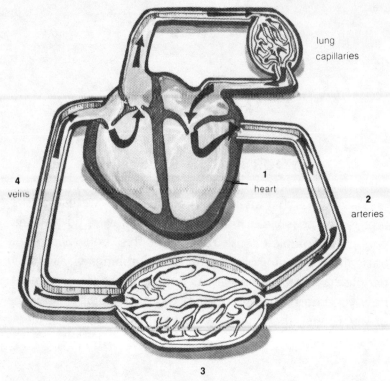

4
veins

1
heart

2
arteries

lung
capillaries

3
body capillaries

This unceasing activity is an important factor in any heart related disorder. The heart is an organ that is in constant motion, expanding and contracting to produce a pumping action. It never rests, except between beats for a fraction of a second, and it thrives on motion. It demands the stimulation of body movement for several reasons, one of which is to prevent the infiltration of fat into the heart muscle, thus hindering its efficient operation. One must keep in motion as much as possible, exercising, walking, going up and down stairs, swimming, dancing, etc. Playing golf on weekends is not sufficient. There must be enough physical activity every single day to increase the heart rate above its normal 68-75 beats per minute. Many cardiologists are of the opinion that 'adequate' exercise means raising the pulse rate to about 120 beats per minute.

THE CIRCULATION: ONE-WAY NETWORK

The network pictured on the preceding page comprises some 60,000 miles of tubing which carries blood to every part of the body. Its most impressive feature is the circular manner in which it keeps the blood moving, always away from the heart in the arteries, toward the heart in the veins — in spite of gravity and in spite of millions of alternate routes. The pump of the heart gives the flow its force, sending freshly oxygenated blood surging out the aorta, the body's largest artery, and into subsidiary arteries, even to the top of the head. The arteries branch out into smaller arterioles, which in turn branch out into millions of microscopic capillaries.

These capillaries eventually unite to form venules, which unite into veins, thin-walled vessels with interior valves which prevent the blood from slipping backward. Thus, the spent blood streams back to the heart. A side trip to the lungs via a pulmonary network refreshes it with oxygen, and it returns to the heart ready to start anew. The entire cycle takes less than a minute.

Exercise is an absolute must for the heart. The heart, like a limb of the body, must get its share of the effect of exercise, otherwise it will lose its tone. Non-exercise of a hand or foot will cause stagnation and atrophy. In a similar fashion the heart loses its ability to respond unless it is in 'shape.'

BLOOD PRESSURE

Blood pressure is given by two figures (example: 120 over 80). It is obtained by inflating a cuff around the upper arm and reducing the compression until it is possible to hear the blood pumping through the blood vessel. When the sound is first heard, it is recorded as the systolic pressure. As the compressium continues to decrease in the cuff, the sound fades away until no longer discernable, the reading at that point is known as the diastolic pressure. The systolic reflects the greatest amount of pressure in the blood vessel — literally during the ejection or pumping phase of the heart, and the diastolic represents the least amount of pressure which occurs during the resting phase of the heart beat.

Although it is impossible to give a normal reading that applies to everyone, a good reading is about 120/80. This should not vary with age to any great degree — an upper normal limit would be 135/90, but I would only consider that normal if the individual were over 65 years of age. Here are a couple of diagnostic tips I have learned over the years which are simple and tell you a great deal about what is going on.

> A Formula to Determine the Work Load of the Heart:
> Multiply pulse rate times the systolic blood pressure.
> Normal is from 8,000 to 9,500.
> If above 9,500 suspect liver, kidney, or athlerosclerosis problems.
> If below 8,000 suspect weak adrenals, weak musculature, vitamin-mineral-protein deficiency.
> If diastolic blood pressure is over 90, suspect liver involvement or sometimes kidney problems.

CONDITIONS WHICH AFFECT BLOOD PRESSURE

We must be aware of the many different conditions which affect blood pressure.

A. STRESS — A spat with your spouse, employer or

children will temporarily raise your blood pressure. So will financial problems, fear and other emotional factors which bring the sympathetic nervous system into play. This sympathetic response will activate the adrenal glands to produce a hormone which tightens up or narrows the diameter of the blood vessels. Physiologically speaking, this is a defense mechanism to enable you to function more efficiently by increasing the amount of oxygen and nutrients available to all tissue cells. Such a temporary increase in blood pressure will not be harmful except if you already have high blood pressure, in which case it could bring about a stroke. This is why chronic hypertensive individuals are always told by their doctor to stay calm and not get too excited.

B. SMOKING — Within seconds after you light up, your blood pressure increases as much as 15-20 points. This action comes from the stimulant effect nicotine has on the adrenal glands which send out a hormone to help defend the body against this deadly toxin. The blood vessels constrict and the pressure goes up!

In the heavy smoker, this constant stimulation with resultant constriction of blood vessels eventually produces a chronic or lasting constriction of the small blood vessels in the extremities. From this we get decreased oxygen and nourishment supply to the areas normally supplied by the capillaries, and a slow degeneration sets in. Eventually a serious, complicated condition known as Buergers Disease can come about. One of the treatments of Buergers Disease is amputation of the limb involved.

C. SODIUM CHLORIDE — Common, ordinary table salt can affect your blood pressure tremendously. We have many chemical balances which normally work in our body to maintain good health. One of these is the 'sodium-potassium pump.' Potassium is a mineral which normally is quite concentrated within the cell and sodium is concentrated in the extra-cellular fluids. These two minerals have a system of alternately bringing nutrients into the cell and discharging wastes from the cell. However if sodium becomes excessive, wastes cannot be discharged from the cell properly and nutrients do not enter it properly.

The extra-cellular fluid increases as does the intra-cellular fluid and a condition known as dropsy or edema occurs. This creates extra pressure on the thousands of miles of blood vessels which automatically increases the pressure inside, resulting in hypertension.

The use of chemical diuretics can bring about this condition by lowering the potassium level. Please note that I am well aware that the common treatment of high blood pressure includes the use of chemical diuretics — in all such cases a great deal of attention should be given to the supplementation of potassium to the diet. The use of diuretics treats one of the symptoms (edema) rather than the cause which is usually a sodium potassium imbalance.

D. KIDNEY DISEASE — Kidney disease brings about hypertension in a similar fashion as a sodium-potassium imbalance would. The kidneys are unable to eliminate the liquid wastes from the body and it accumulates, producing edema. Excessive smoking, a high carbohydrate diet and excessive coffee and tea drinking are all contributing factors to kidney disease.

E. LIVER CONGESTION — All the blood in the body flows through the liver, both for detoxification and to pick up nutrients which the liver stores. If the liver is congested with toxins or chemicals, overriden with fatty degeneration, or has lost its ability to function properly because of continual abuse by alcohol and has become hardened, a back pressure builds up in the portal circulation which can be reflected in the whole body circulation as hypertension. It has been my experience that liver congestion is the most common cause of high blood pressure, and my contention is backed by hundreds of patients who no longer suffer from hypertension as a result of treatment directed at restoring liver function.

F. ATHEROSCLEROSIS-ARTERIOSCLEROSIS — We will not overlook what many feel is the cause of high blood pressure — the narrowing of the arterial system by deposits of calcium, cholesterol, fibrin, and other blood constituents in what is commonly referred to as atherosclerosis or arteriosclerosis. I will respectfully offer an opinion that we have the old question here: what came first — the chicken or the egg? Or, in more appropriate context — liver congestion or atherosclerosis. Liver congestion can produce high blood pressure as outlined before, high blood pressure can cause eddy currents and erosion of the wall of the artery which the constituents of the blood stream tried to 'patch up' by forming a barricade so that the blood would not leak out. It has been scientifically determined that, in a cholesterol plaque which forms on the wall of an artery, the first part laid down is fibrin which is a blood protein acting to form clots because of its peculiar 'fish net' appearance. After that the calcium, cholesterol, other blood proteins, triglycerides, etc. seem to attach themselves to this 'net' and the plaque is formed. I am of the firm opinion that cholesterol is *not* the *cause* of atherosclerosis. (For further information on the subject see the chapter on the subject of cholesterol).

It should be noted that the substance known as lecithin has the ability to keep blood fats (cholesterol, triglycerides, etc.) in solution in the blood stream because it makes their surfaces 'slippery' and they do not clump together forming clots or plaques.

G. TUMORS — In a very small proportion of high blood pressure patients other factors such as tumors are involved. Most of these are really surgical cases and do not properly come under this discussion.

NOW I KNOW WHY, BUT . . .

Perhaps more are interested in knowing what to do about high blood pressure rather than its causes. I must begin by saying that it is important to understand the seriousness of the condition to properly be motivated to eliminate the cause. Study the following charts and understand the impact that your blood pressure can have on your life.

CAUSES & CURES

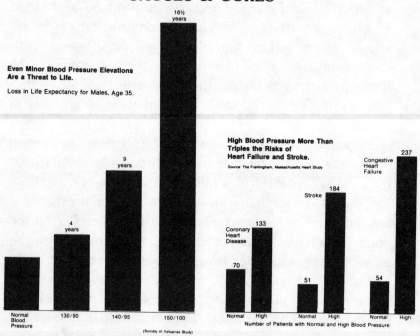

Even Minor Blood Pressure Elevations Are a Threat to Life.

Loss in Life Expectancy for Males, Age 35.

16½ years

9 years

4 years

Normal Blood Pressure | 130/90 | 140/95 | 150/100

(Society of Actuaries Study)

High Blood Pressure More Than Triples the Risks of Heart Failure and Stroke.

Source: The Framingham, Massachusetts Heart Study

Coronary Heart Disease — Normal 70, High 133

Stroke — Normal 51, High 184

Congestive Heart Failure — Normal 54, High 237

Number of Patients with Normal and High Blood Pressure

A. STRESS — We discussed stress as being a factor in hypertension — although not a major one, in my opinion. Unless the stress is continuous, it will not create the sustained, dangerous high blood pressure which kills or cripples. Adequate rest — at least eight hours of sleep each night often helps in relieving tension, as does a good nutritional program. We have outlined such a program at the end of this book under "Creative Restoration Diet." Many will find that in addition to a good diet, a complete vitamin and mineral supplement works miracles in restoring body chemistry to better accommodate the stress of daily living without becoming hypertensive.

B. SMOKING — The effect of smoking is dramatic on the blood vascular tree. But how can one stop without going through the agonies of withdrawal so common to drugs? Few are able to 'cold turkey' stop smoking — the change is so abrupt and causes such an inner craving that help is needed. My advice is to follow this program.

1. Eat at least 6 small meals per day even if you are not hungry.
2. Eat primarily proteins (meat, milk, eggs, fish, nuts, seeds), with a moderate amount of fat containing food such as cream, butter, oil in salad dressing, etc.
3. Snack on raw vegetables all you wish.
4. Avoid carbohydrates (sugar containing foods) as if they were the plague.
5. Find some kind of physical exercise that you enjoy and indulge in it every day.
6. Use a complete vitamin and mineral supplement similar to the recommended formula at the end of this chapter.

This program will restore normal body chemistry and keep a constant blood sugar level which will prevent the headaches, tremors and other withdrawal symptoms.

C. SODIUM CHLORIDE — Since the use of sodium chloride is a definite factor in high blood pressure, I highly suggest that you eliminate it completely from your kitchen cupboard. Many are able to enjoy the flavor of food without the use of this substance and have no difficulty in adapting. Some may feel they wish to use a flavoring or seasoning agent, and for them I suggest the following:

1. Herb seasonings including kelp, etc. Be sure and read the label so that the product you purchase is not predominately sodium chloride.

2. A mixture of potassium and sodium chloride (approx. 60% potassium and 40% sodium chloride) is now on the market. This is very salty to the taste, and because of the amount of potassium contained prevents the water retention we discussed previously as a causative factor in hypertension.

Under no circumstances use 'sea salt' or 'earth salt' as these are primarily sodium chloride.

D. KIDNEY DISEASE — Although there are a variety of kidney diseases, all of them are benefitted by an increased consumption of fluids, particularly water. It is suggested that *all* coffee, tea, alcohol and high sugar containing beverages be discontinued if you have kidney disease. You may have to force yourself to drink water for a short period, but soon you will find that you prefer this 'universal solvent.' Some may wish to drink distilled water; if you do so be sure to supplement with a broad spectrum mineral such as found in the formula at the end of this chapter. I do not recommend using tap water unless it is good spring or well water without contaminants. Many have found the use of filtered water a convenient way to solve this situation. Under the sink units, attached to the faucet units, and portable units are available from your local health food store.

The use of the Liver Kidney Cleansing Fast outlined later is an excellent means of restoring kidney function. Try it!

E. LIVER CONGESTION — This is, in my opinion, the most prevalent cause of hypertension. In order to decongest the liver, it is necessary to abstain from food for a few days. The Liver-Kidney Cleansing Fast outlined later is an absolute must for any patient who wishes to see results fast in hypertension. Since the program is detailed later, I will not enlarge here but after you are off the fast, I suggest you use some herbs to create a continuation of the cleansing process. Herbs are nature's medicines and are very effective in accomplishing cleansing throughout the body. I use a combination of several herbs, all of which have complimentary cleansing properties: Garlic, Mandrake, Quassia, Black Cohosh, Chaparral, Foenugreek, Red Sage and Golden Seal. This combination is available as a single tablet from your health food store.

The use of some of these, such as garlic, have a long-term use in folk medicine for the treatment of high blood pressure, and have withstood the test of time. These are rather inexpensive and can be purchased from your local health food store. The importance of this continued cleansing cannot be emphasized too much — in hypertension there are degenerative changes which have taken place and the liver is the single most important organ in re-establishing normal body chemistry.

After completing the cleansing fast, your next step is to use the Creative Restoration Diet as your guideline in eating habits for the rest of your life. It is an enjoyable, healthy way to choose and combine foods.

Regarding supplements, the B-Complex vitamins will help to hasten the recovery of your liver, as well as provide insurance against future occurrences. It is my opinion that the B-Complex factors should be taken in combination with a total vitamin-mineral supplement for best results.

F. ARTERIOSCLEROSIS-ATHEROSCLEROSIS

Since a decrease in the diameter of a blood vessel will produce high blood pressure, we should explore means of reducing such accumulations inside the walls of the arteries.

1. CHELATION — This is a method of introducing into the blood stream a synthetic amino acid, which has

the chemical property of binding deposited calcium and other minerals and carrying it out of the body via the urine. When the minerals are picked up from the blood vessel wall, they disrupt the other accumulated materials (cholesterol, etc.) and thus clear the channel and automatically lower the blood pressure because of a larger diameter in the artery. Check your local health food store for a doctor who uses this procedure. Chelation offers a new direction for hope in advanced hardening of the arteries since it influences the basic pathology taking place. The surgical procedure to replace arteries do not in any way stop the disease process progression in other areas of the body.

2. AMINO ACID CHELATED MINERALS — The use of amino acid chelated minerals orally can accomplish a similar effect in less serious cases, but it takes

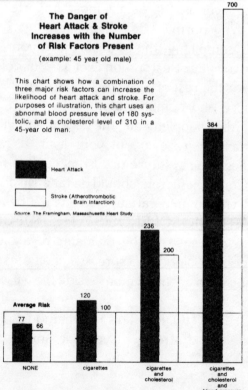

The Danger of Heart Attack & Stroke Increases with the Number of Risk Factors Present

(example: 45 year old male)

This chart shows how a combination of three major risk factors can increase the likelihood of heart attack and stroke. For purposes of illustration, this chart uses an abnormal blood pressure level of 180 systolic, and a cholesterol level of 310 in a 45-year old man.

■ Heart Attack

□ Stroke (Atherothrombotic Brain Infarction)

Source: The Framingham, Massachusetts Heart Study

longer. I have indicated a formula which is generally proper for such use in the end of this chapter. Although some would like to be very specific in the use of single amino acid chelates, the broad spectrum of minerals is the best for this use in that no imbalances occur in the blood stream.

G. TUMORS — A tumor of the kidneys or adrenal can cause hypertension. These are usually non-malignant and are the cause of only a very few cases of high blood pressure. The surgical removal of such tumor will relieve the blood pressure and a proper diet and supplement program can help prevent such a recurrence.

SYNOPSIS

If you wish to overcome hypertension the following program is a must:

1. Stop smoking.
2. Don't drink coffee, tea, alcohol, cola drinks, or high sugar beverages.
3. Don't use common table salt. Substitute herbs or a combination potassium-sodium salt.
4. Do drink lots of water — about 2 quarts daily.
5. Use the Liver-Kidney Cleansing Diet.
6. Follow the cleansing by adhering to the Creative Restoration Diet as your food guidelines.
7. If you have hypertension complicated with arterio-sclerosis or atherosclerosis, it might be worth your while to consider chelation therapy from a physician to cleanse your arteries.
8. To support all body functions, their restoration to normal and the maintenance of these functions, use a broad spectrum vitamin and mineral supplement program.

9. Apply the principles of botanical medicine by using herbs to assist in cleansing the liver. Once your desired blood pressure has been reached, you can discontinue such preparations but the periodic use (30 days every 6 months) is good prevention.

SAMPLE FORMULA OF A BALANCED VITAMIN-MINERAL COMPLEX

Vitamin A .... 25,000 IU	Inositol 60mg
Vitamin D 400IU	Folic Acid 400mcg
Vitamin E 400IU	Biotin 100mcg
Vitamin C 1,200mg	Calcium 1000mg
Vitamin B-1 .... 60mg	Magnesium 400mg
Vitamin B-2 .... 60mg	Phosphorus 150mg
Vitamin B-6 .... 60mg	Potassium 99mg
Vitamin B-12 .... 100mcg	Iron 15mg
Niacin 30mg	Iodine .... 225 mcg
Niacinamide 30mg	Copper 2mg
Pantothenic Acid 100mg	Chromium .... 500 mcg
PABA 60mg	Manganese 15mg
Choline 60mg	Zinc 15mg

SAMPLE FORMULA OF AMINO ACID CHELATED MULTI-MINERAL

Calcium	375mg
Phosphorus	75mg
Magnesium	180mg
Iodine	225mcg
Iron	15mg
Copper	3mg
Zinc	15mg
Chromium	200mcg
Potassium	99mg
Manganese	30mg
Selenium	20mcg

LOW BLOOD PRESSURE

There has been much said about high blood pressure, but what about low blood pressure? It is often considered insignificant by the physician on examination because surely this patient will not die from a stroke and very rarely if ever has arterio or atherosclerosis. To the victim, it does mean they have less energy than they would like, they often have poor adaptive mechanism to a drop in environmental temperature, and they sometimes note that they get dizzy easily when changing from a sitting or reclining position to an upright stance. The dizziness and other symptoms are usually from a lack of oxygen to the brain or other extremities from low blood pressure.

This condition is almost always related to low functioning adrenal glands and is best overcome by using various means to restore the adrenals. Proper diet as outlined in the Creative Restoration Diet is essential. The use of a good multi-vitamin-mineral complex is also necessary. For difficult cases you will want to add extra pantothenic acid for a total daily intake of 3,000 mg., extra vitamin C for a total of 4,000 mg. daily, and extra potassium for a total of 1,500 mg. daily. For those who are interested in an all out program, I would suggest the addition of vitamin E to this program in the amount of approximately 1,000 IU daily, as this decreases the body's need for oxygen.

Another very important adjunct is the use of glandular DNA (deoxyribonucleic acid) factors to assist nature in rebuilding new cells. These are cellular blueprints which have the formula for specific ingredients needed to rebuild a cell when it is worn out and dies. We often find multiple glandular involvement, so the use of a multiple glandular extract is superior to targeting in on a single gland. The entire glandular system is rejuvenated and balanced out

241

when a multiple extract is used. These substances are often referred to as nucleoproteins and are found in health food stores.

This nucleo-protein-vitamin-mineral approach is the most effective I know in alleviating low blood pressure.

SAMPLE FORMULA OF NUCLEO PROTEIN

Adrenal 60mg
Pituitary 10mg
Heart 60mg
Kidney 60mg
Thymus 60mg
Pancreas 60mg
RNA 40mg

Chapter 16

AFTER HYSTERECTOMY

So you've had a hysterectomy — like thousands of other women. There is no use crying over spilled milk, but there is much value in critical evaluation and self-appraisal. You are now a changed woman, but the world has not come to an end! There is much you can do. First of all, what happened to you?

WHAT IS A HYSTERECTOMY?

Very simply, the term hysterectomy refers to the surgical removal of the uterus or womb. There are different types, so let's review them:

1. Simple Hysterectomy — Only the uterus is removed.
2. Total Hysterectomy — The cervix is removed along with the uterus.
3. Pan-Total Hysterectomy — Removal of uterus, cervix, tubes and ovaries.

For your own information you might wish to ask your doctor what kind of procedure was performed on you. It will help you to understand more thoroughly and apply the information which follows.

HOW ARE YOU NOW DIFFERENT?

This is a very basic question that must be faced before proceeding with any sort of realistic life program. One thing for sure is that you are no longer capable of having a baby. That is a thing of the past, and there is absolutely no remedy. If you have had a simple hysterectomy and still have your own ovaries, it means that about the only kind of difference you will experience is that you will no longer have any menstrual periods. There will usually be no hormonal imbalances to contend with and there is neither physical nor hormonal interferences with your sex life. Everything should be "normal" except for the lack of periods.

However, under certain circumstances there are hormonal changes even when the ovaries are not removed. Hot flashes, emotional disturbances and other symptoms of menopause appear as if the ovaries were removed. After discussing this with surgeons, the most logical answer seems to be that certain blood supply routes to the ovaries are severed by the surgery so the ovaries are literally isolated from normal blood supply carrying nutrients to the cells and waste products away. This, of course, leads to malfunction. The management procedure, when this occurs, should be just the same as if the ovaries were removed.

Complications arise when the ovaries have been removed, you are now in INSTANT MENOPAUSE. During normal life patterns, the ovaries came into importance when you began having periods. Remember how your thought patterns changed during those years? Your attitudes toward all sorts of things, including boys, suddenly took a different light.

The activity of the ovaries did this to you through their hormonal actions. You also developed physically insofar as your body was concerned — hips, shoulders, thighs, tilt of the pelvis, breasts and a multitude of other physical and functional characteristics. You do not lose these features now that the ovaries are gone, but the power that developed them is gone. In a sense, it is the use of these features that is altered, not that they are absent. For instance, you need not have a changed sex life because of your hysterectomy, but you will lack the cyclic hormonal influences you've had these many years.

Your ovaries also maintained a degree of influence over the metabolism of the body; the fullness of your skin, muscle tone, sharpness of thought, appetite for life and much more. They are being altered. The variation is in the direction of aging. In one sense, it is the activity of the ovaries that tend to delay the aging process. The longer and stronger your ovaries produce in normal life, the younger you stay as the years keep rolling along. During the usual life pattern, decline of ovarian function comes on gradually. It is hardly perceptible until it is there. Your surgical menopause was not gradual, but instant. Suddenly you no longer had the bodily influence of the ovarian hormones and yet the body was forced to carry on with an alternate plan of action, unprepared though it may have been.

Another factor to remember is that this INSTANT MENOPAUSE has varying degrees of influence on you depending where you are in the normal pattern of declining life. Are you in your prime years or beyond? The younger you are, the more dramatic the change from normal hormonal activity to the alternate state.

PHYSIOLOGICAL CHANGES

To be more specific about the hormonal activities of the ovaries, one must mention that the ovaries normally produce two types of hormones: estrogens and progesterones. The normal functions of these hormones are:

1. To maintain estrus (menstrual cycle).
2. To prepare the uterus and body for pregnancy.
3. To develop and maintain female characteristics: voice pattern, temperament, attitudes, body shape (hips, shoulders, thighs, etc.), breast development and other sexual individualities.

Estrogen is more active during the first half of the monthly cycle though present up until just before menses. It tends to rebuild the endometrial (inside) lining of the uterus. It also causes the follicle (egg sac) to ripen, ready for ovulation.

Progesterone starts its effect by causing ovulation or release of the ovum from the follicle and processing the endometrium to make it ready for implantation of the fertilized ovum. It works until just before menses. Menses occurs when both estrogens and progesterones drop to minimal levels.

PSYCHOLOGICAL CHANGES

Obviously, there are physical changes which occur on a cyclical basis. There are associated emotional or psychological changes which are normal for the various phases of the cycle. However, the emotional phases can become more than they should be when compounded by other stresses in a woman's life. Outside stresses make her much more susceptible to the inevitable cyclic stresses of estrus.

Now that you no longer have ovaries you are not a candidate for the cyclic stresses but you are a victim of having no ovarian hormones, except for a small amount secreted by the adrenals which is grossly insufficient as compared to ovarian secretion. You now miss many of the systemic subtleties which have no apparent connection to ovarian function. Not only are there mood changes, concentration difficulties and other psychological reactions, but also problems with the system which controls your blood vessels: you have hot flashes.

To understand hot flashes one must reassess the overall picture:

1. The ovaries have been surgically removed.
2. There has been a sudden or instant cessation of ovarian hormonal activity, INSTANT MENOPAUSE.
3. The thyroid and adrenal glands had no warning that such would happen, as would occur in a natural menopause.
4. Such a reaction is a severe stress which shows itself in the strained reaction of the adrenal cortex.
5. Also, the thyroid is stressed so that it may and probably will work abnormally for a period of time.
6. These combined ovarian, adrenal and thyroid reactions cause an instability of the control mechanism governing your circulation with resultant temporary flushing or hot flashes.
7. The same sort of picture can develop in the normal menopause but one can question how "normal" such a reaction is even though it is common. Actually, "ideal" is normal and "ideal" does not include control mechanisms which don't work. Hot flashes, in the after-hysterectomy woman, are the result of absent ovaries with stressed thyroid and adrenal glands. It is a multiglandular dysfunction.

Keep these concepts in mind when thinking about the INSTANT MENOPAUSE — several glands are involved and should be supported by multiglandular therapy.

ALTERNATE MECHANISM

Normally, the body has a built-in alternative mechanism

247

to be used in the transition from full activity to the alternative. First, there is a gradual decline in ovarian function which lessens the shock of sudden cessation or INSTANT MENOPAUSE. Second, there are other sources of ovarian hormones in the body — the adrenal cortex glands. They have been producing hormones similar to those produced by the ovaries all these years without your knowing it.

The amount produced is only a small percentage of the total capability of your own ovaries when in the prime. But now, when the menopause is coming, this small percentage becomes a nice figure in reserve. It is a life saver which protects you from the effects of total hormone withdrawal. It is even helping you now since you have attained INSTANT MENOPAUSE. The degree of help will vary individually since you are unique in yourself. It will also vary in effect because of your own circumstances.

1. What was the situation in your life before surgery?
2. What was the surgical procedure like and its effect on your body?
3. What were the anesthetic and post-anesthetic effects on your body?
4. What were the post-operative medications and how have your reacted subsequently to all these new variables (stresses) and to your changed life?

STRESS FACTORS

All of these are bare facts of life in how your body will respond to its current status. One thing in common is that they are all stress factors. Stress is always a drain on the adrenal cortex glands since the adrenal glands are the headquarters for anti-stress activity within the body. Were your adrenal glands in good shape before all this happened, or were you on the verge of emotional problems or other physical problems? If so, then you can expect even more severe symptoms resulting from the INSTANT MENO-PAUSE. Regardless, the current stress is one to contend with and deserves your total attention. It means a change in life style patterns, at least for a while.

Remember, no one else can make these decisions for you. It is your body and you are now in charge of what your body is to do and what it will receive. Unfortunately, you do not have the liberty of leisure during which you can do all the reading on the subject you may want to do. If you talk to the doctor, he will give you a more or less standard sort of answer about the usage of hormone substitution therapy and enough sedation to compensate for some of the bad times ahead. With this you have another immediate problem — are the synthetic hormones carcinogenic? "Will I get cancer if I take them?" This is a very real problem. "If the hormone withdrawal symptoms from the INSTANT MENOPAUSE are severe, do I take the risk of cancer or don't I? What are the relative factors to consider?

These are questions and decisions you must make almost immediately, even, it may seem, almost before you recover from the anesthetic.

NUTRITIONAL THERAPY

There are some alternate courses of action that deserve consideration. They work and should be investigated. Yet, there is little time for procrastination. You should have been presented these factors for consideration even before your surgery. The odds are a thousand to one that you were not given even a hint that there were some sort of alternate choices. Ironically, it is possible that such choices made presurgically might have eliminated the need for surgery entirely.

VITAMIN E

The first consideration is vitamin E. This is a very controversial substance. (Incidentally, controversial drugs are not controversial or obsolete because of effectiveness versus non-effectiveness. They simply are caught up in political battle.) There is no doubt in my mind that vitamin E is reasonably effective in the menopause. It should be in the form of mixed tocopherols and rated as d-alpha in international units. Some recent work indicates that a dosage of upwards to 1000 IU daily may be needed to allay menopausal symptoms. For this reason, this substance should have prime consideration in lessening the symptoms resultant from INSTANT MENOPAUSE. Vitamin E should always be used with wisdom. Certainly, do not start with the maximum dosage until you discover what you can or cannot achieve on lesser dosages. Start with about 400 IU daily, then, gradually, increase the dosage as indicated. The one possible bad effect that demands alertness is an increase in blood pressure. Certainly, this does not occur in any more than a very small percentage of vitamin E users, but to them it can be very important. Judicious use can overcome this threat.

MINERALS

The next order of business is to balance the minerals in your body. This is called homeostasis — where all the various minerals are balanced between and among each other. It is a multi-faceted situation. Calcium is the one to consider first. A normal body needs about 1000 mg. daily. It is quite possible that your body now in INSTANT MENOPAUSE, may need more than this suggested intake. As regards intake and absorption of calcium, there is apparently little difference in the source of the calcium since the acidity in the stomach breaks the bonds of the compound so that the ionized form is passed into the duodenum. This ionized form is then chelated in the duodenum and absorbed into the system. Chelation is the process of covering minerals with an amino acid cover to make them more readily assimilable. It would appear that 2000 mg. daily would be sufficient for the usual after-hysterectomy woman.

Phosphorus should be provided in a ratio of about 1 part phosphorus to 2½ parts calcium, or 800 mg. phosphorus for 2000 mg. calcium.

Finally, calcium metabolism cannot proceed properly without sufficiency of hydrochloric acid, HCl, which is harder to come by in the older age group. Hydrochloric acid is available in health food stores as Betaine Hydrochloride.

MAGNESIUM

Magnesium is very important to body metabolism. It is involved in upwards to 70% of all enzyme systems in the body. It is therefore only logical to assist the body to metabolize normally by supplying adequacy of magnesium.

Magnesium is available in many forms, magnesium carbonate, magnesium oxide, magnesium gluconate, magnesium chloride, etc. Excess intake will cause a laxative effect (epsom salts is magnesium sulfate), but when properly combined with other minerals, this very rarely occurs. The need for magnesium is so urgent that certain medical researchers have administered magnesium intravenously with immediate and dramatic results.

Magnesium interacts with calcium specifically to relax and calm the nerves and muscles — in fact, is so effective that it has been called the "lullaby" mineral. The importance of this mineral cannot be overemphasized, both because of its enzyme involvement and its relaxant effects.

TRACE MINERALS

Trace minerals are important factors in good health and are found in raw vegetables, fruits, nuts and seeds. Also, a good multimineral tablet will be very beneficial to insure adequate supply.

NUTRIENTS FRIENDLY TO THE NERVES

As you are well aware, your nerves are involved in this whole picture. Nerves control every action of the body. You have been through a lot of experiences where your nerves have been abused to the maximum. It is only logical to support them by providing their "favorite nutrients" and to soothe them any way possible. They do not suffer from a deficiency of 'Valium'®.

VITAMIN B COMPLEX

Incidentally, one of the friendly nerve nutrients is the vitamin B complex. This is a whole complex containing all of the B factors plus the naturally associated synergistic micro-nutrients. B complex includes B-1 (Thiamin), B-2 (Riboflavin), B-3 (Niacin, Niacinamide), B-6 (Pyridoxine), Choline, Inositol, PABA, Pantothenic acid, B-12 (Cyanocobalamin), Biotin, Folic Acid and others.

Synergistic micronutrients consist of minerals, enzymes, DNA, RNA, and many sub-molecular and sub-atomic factors about which we know very little. They are important because they provide the body with necessary ingredients so the vitamin can be metabolized entirely without robbing the body of other needed nutritional stores. The B complex family is usually found in cereals, nuts, and organ meats.

Supplements containing B complex can be in comparatively large amounts providing that the synergistic micronutrients in the form of yeast or rice bran are provided in the base material.

LIPIDS

Lipids are the fats in our food supply — they may be saturated or unsaturated depending on their source. These fats break down to cholesterol, triglycerides, phospholipids and are extensively utilized throughout the body. Many are not aware of the important part that cholesterol plays in normal nerve transmission, or in vitamin D conversion from ultraviolet light. These fats also form the basis of hormones which control so many of the functions of the body. So, let us emphasize that the presence of fats or lipids in our diet is extremely important. Unfortunately good lipids are not easy to come by in modern diets. Avocados, fresh nuts, fertile eggs and raw cream are excellent sources. The essential fatty acids should be included in the above regimen. Highly processed, man-made lipids, particularly the hydrogenated oils such as margarine and homogenized milk, are particularly detrimental and should never be consumed.

PROTEIN

Proteins are the basic building blocks of the body structure. Our whole body has a protein framework. Proteins are also the basis for enzymes and some of the hormones. As such, it becomes obvious that protein in the dietary is not to be considered lightly. Both quantity and quality are essential factors. Some amino acids, the constituents of proteins, are called essential because they cannot be manufactured within the body. Others are non-essential but are needed as a quantity factor. They all work together under the influence of DNA—RNA, hormones and enzymes to become the body framework or to be used for energy production.

In the INSTANT MENOPAUSAL woman, proteins are particularly important because of the immediate post-operative need for tissue repair and healing. They are also important because the immediate lack of hormones definitely hinders protein metabolism and the body can not keep up its repair and maintenance standards. The body tends to deteriorate more rapidly. Also, protein provides strong chelating agents, the amino acids, needed for proper mineral absorption. Finally, the potential lack of adequate hydrochloric acid in the stomach hastens body decline because of decreased protein digestion. In particular, protein will help you heal and maintain your adrenals and nervous system as well as provide the basic amino acids needed to make hormones, in your case: corticosterioids, estrogens and progesterones as produced by the adrenal cortex. Since you no longer have ovaries, the adrenal cortex glands become "super important" for you.

DNA-RNA

Other factors which are very important in the support of the nervous system as well as the adrenals are the DNA and RNA intra-nuclear factors. These are found respectively in special tissue extracts and concentrates which are processed in the raw state to preserve all the naturally associated synergistic micro-nutrients.

The action of these substances is to normalize the tissues corresponding to the source; i.e., adrenal for adrenal, lung for lung, etc. Some may claim ineffectiveness since they are digested in the stomach when taken by mouth. True, they are digested but the proper composite of amino acids becomes present in the blood after absorption so that the tissue itself can more easily glean sufficiency for rebuilding its own tissue. It works and is non-toxic. Excesses of DNA-RNA in the dietary are simply utilized as ordinary protein without any undue consequence. In your situation, your nerves and the entire glandular system, particularly the adrenals, certainly deserve all the friendly support available. For the glands, a multiglandular approach is more logical; i.e. support them all.

VITAMIN C

Vitamin C is used by every cell of the body, but particularly the adrenocortical cells. Vitamin C is ultimately concerned with collagen metabolism which is the basic protein structure of the body. It, also, is involved with cementum, the substance holding cells in capillaries together. In your case, it's particularly important because of the adrenocortical influence.

In extreme cases of avitaminosis C, there are splinter-type hemorrhages in the adrenal cortex glands, called Waterhouse-Fredrickson's Disease. Actually, the hemorrhages destroy the very cells that would utilize the vitamin C to protect the body. These hemorrhages are also noted in cortisone therapy evidencing some of the abuse to the adrenal cortex by these medications. Mega C dosages are certainly indicated at any time the adrenocortical glands are stressed. In our society, our need is every day; but with you, who are suffering the INSTANT MENOPAUSE, it is every day plus, plus. This means you must mega-C supplement your body if you wish any semblance of normalcy.

PANTOTHENIC ACID

Another vitamin specially concerned with adrenocortical function is pantothenic acid. Symptoms of deficiency are usually slow and vague, like headache, malaise, nausea, occasional vomiting accompanied by flatus, cramping in abdomen and legs, loss of antibody production and impaired motor coordination. There is a definite loss of stamina and integrity of the individual which is really just a reflection of the failure of the adrenal glands. Pantothenic acid and niacin are both used synergistically with ACTH (adrenocorticotrophic hormone from the pituitary) in the substance used by the body to combat stress. Lack of pantothenic acid means devoid of anti-stress action by the adrenal glands.

VITAMIN A

Whenever resistance or defense is in question, one vitamin which comes to the forefront is vitamin A. Due to the extra demands made upon the system to maintain itself, it may be wise to include vitamin A in the armamentarium in dosages from 50,000 to 200,000 I.U. daily. This may sound huge to you and you may be warned by some more conservative persons who really do not know from practical experience that such dosages are very valuable, yet innocuous and not dangerous. Symptoms like peeling skin and loss of hair can occur with much larger dosages. Even so, they are only temporary drawbacks and not permanent problems as one finds with toxic drugs.

ADRENALS

As you noted throughout this whole discussion, the

adrenals are repeatedly mentioned. They are important to you because they are the anti-stress headquarters for the body and you certainly are under stress. Secondly, they are now your only internal source of estrogens and progesterones. As such they should be treated with T.L.C. Every nutritional suggestion mentioned herein has the adrenal gland in view and you should too.

EXERCISE

Another factor which is not nutritionally oriented but is holistically important, is exercise. You should have planned exercises performed on a daily basis. It neither has to be a marathon-type nor a back-breaking episode. It must be the simple utilization of your body on a daily basis. Keep active and you will stimulate your circulation, lymph drainage, and keep the muscles in trim. It is just plain common sense. Swimming, walking, jogging, running, rope jumping are considered excellent types of exercise.

SUMMARY

INSTANT MENOPAUSE need not be the living hell that many women go through. The following is a summary of the procedure suggested by the author as a common sense program of assisting the body to retain and maintain as near normal function as possible.

1. Follow the Creative Restoration Diet very closely as an every day eating pattern.
2. Incorporate exercise into every day of your life. If you value your good health, this is an absolute must — regardless of age.

257

3. Use a good multi-vitamin-mineral formulation similar to the one listed below every day.

SAMPLE FORMULA OF A BALANCED VITAMIN-MINERAL COMPLEX

Vitamin A	25,000IU	Folic Acid	40mcg
Vitamin D	400IU	Biotin	100mcg
Vitamin E	400IU	Calcium	1,000mg
Vitamin C	1,200mg	Magnesium	400mg
Vitamin B-1	60mg	Phosphorus	150mg
Vitamin B-2	60mg	Potassium	99mg
Vitamin B-6	60mg	Iron	15mg
Vitamin B-12	100mcg	Iodine	225mcg
Niacin	30mg	Copper	2mg
Niacinamide	30mg	Chromium	200mcg
Pantothenic Acid	100mg	Manganese	15mg
PABA	60mg	Selenium	100mcg
Choline	60mg	Zinc	15mg
Inositol	60mg		

4. Add extra vitamin E — up to a total of 2,000 I.U. per day depending on how much it takes to equalize your circulation.

5. The use of a multiglandular extract similar to the following can have an excellent effect on glandular normalization. Your body functions as a total organism not a series of parts. A multiglandular DNA-RNA preparation tends to support a function of the body from its different aspects thus acting in a more normal manner than one could accomplish with singular glandulars.

Ovarian Substance	60mg
Whole Pituitary Substance	20mg
Adrenal Substance	60mg
Thymus Substance	60mg
Pancreas Substance	60mg
Kidney Substance	60mg
Heart Substance	60mg
Ribonucleic Acid (RNA)	60mg

6. You may wish to increase your iodine intake as described herein. Your metabolic rate stabilizes when you do.

If we can say in just a few words our feeling on this artificially created condition, it would be extremely encouraging because we have seen so many women regain comparative normalcy by following these procedures.

DIETARY

Finally, comes the dietary. This will be discussed in detail in the Creative Restoration Diet.

Chapter 17

INDIGESTION

You must be one of the millions of Americans who suffer from some sort of problem with their digestive tract. Since TV advertising has a high percentage of ads concerning antacids and other substances for indigestion, you must know full well that you are not alone — in fact, there are enough of you to support this fantastic advertising budget as well as providing profits for the advertisers.

So let's take a closer look.

The digestive tract is a tube of the outside world passing through our bodies. It starts at the lips and ends with the anus. Its purpose is to provide for the intake and digestion of food, the absorption of nutrients, and the excretion of waste materials. When the digestive tract functions well, good health usually follows. When the digestive tract does not function normally, many different things can go wrong.

BURP AND BELCH

When a person burps and belches, it means that the digestive function is not normal. Something has gone wrong in the food processing department. It is primarily a stomach problem. The stomach is where the body begins digesting the protein found in food. Pepsin is the main digesting

261

enzyme secreted by the stomach and is activated by hydrochloric acid which is also secreted by the stomach. The two work together to start digesting protein. When there is an insufficiency of hydrochloric acid in the stomach, protein is not digested according to schedule and gas forms which becomes the burp and belch.

When protein is slow in being digested, the carbohydrates in the stomach tend to ferment (a bacterial process) and form the gas which is so symptomatic. It is a kind of mismatch when we consume concentrated carbohydrates with concentrated proteins, since the carbohydrates really don't need to stay in the stomach for any length of time at all. They are not digested in the stomach but pass quickly into the small intestine if consumed alone. On the other hand, if they are consumed with concentrated protein, most of them are trapped in the stomach while protein waits to be digested, even up to five hours. A low level of hydrochloric acid further compounds the problem since a normal or high level would inhibit fermentation in the stomach. (Hydrochloric acid kills bacteria).

A simple remedy for this condition is to improve your digestive capability by taking a digest aid tablet, which contains hydrochloric acid and pepsin. A test to see if you need digest aids is to take five tablets of such a product with a meal. If you do not suffer from the usual burps and belches, you have proven in one hour that you have need for digestive support. If five tablets solve your problems, try four with the next meal. If four still solves the belching and burping, then try three. By gradually reducing the dosage of the digest aids, you will finally have a recurrence of the old symptoms of burping and belching. At this low point, slowly increase the dosage each meal to find what is the dosage you need to prevent symptoms. Continue that dosage indefinitely so long as you do not develop hyperacidity or heartburn, which is nothing more than a burning sensation in the stomach. If heartburn develops, it tells you the current dosage is too high. The proper dosage relieves your old symptoms and does not create new ones.

It is a good rule of thumb when planning your meals to consider eating fruits and vegetables together; meats, dairy products, fish, etc., with vegetables but not with fruits, fruit juices or other concentrated sweets. Such a rule is very effective in helping to control some discomfort, and with the addition of a digestive aid, you can have a trouble-free digestion.

HEARTBURN AND HYPERACIDITY

Antacid advertising has made you an expert on the mechanism of antacid therapy. Unfortunately, commercial advertising is not revealing the total picture. In the first place, heartburn is a late manifestation of the problem. At first, there is not enough hydrochloric acid in the stomach so that the emptying time may be delayed. When the delay is rather prolonged, some bile is regurgitated or backflowed from the duodenum (the next part of the digestive tract), back into the stomach. Bile is very irritative and caustic. It can cause the stomach lining to become irritated, angry and even ulcerated. The alkaline nature of the bile causes reflex secretion of hydrochloric acid so that the food is then churned and digested by pepsin and hydrochloric acid so the stomach empties. In essence this means that the stomach only becomes hyperacidic after the bile has been regurgitated into the stomach. There was too little in the first place, now there is too much. It is not a matter of acid concentration because normal pH can be as high as one (the strongest acid). It is the matter of how much (quantity) of acid secreted. More acid acts for a longer period of time. It is also a matter of timing of acid secretion into the stomach. Many times, heartburn victims have acid secretion at night time when the stomach may already be empty.

The irritation to the gastric mucous membrane by the bile and late acid secretion causes contraction of the small arteries in the stomach wall called arteriolar spasm. This results in reduced integrity of the stomach wall so that the alkaline reaction of the bile and the acid reaction of the hydrochloric acid alternately act to erode the stomach mucosa. Before an open ulcer develops there would be irritation or gastritis which was preceded by heartburn or hyperacidity. Big problems always start small.

Nutritional care of such a condition includes a nonirritating high protein diet including predigested protein and raw pancreatic DNA-RNA. Take a level teaspoonful or four tablets of the raw pancreatic concentrate and chew it thoroughly at least four times daily. Use oftener to control pain if symptoms occur before a scheduled dose. Do not allow pain to develop. Well chewed almonds can also assist, as do raw cream, avocados and non-flavored full-fat yogurt. One can live on such a diet for a month or more if necessary to allow healing to take place. It should take about four to six weeks to heal an ulcer crater. You should be without distress shortly after starting such a program, but the healing still takes a long time.

BLOATING

Bloating is the after-meal collection of upper intestinal gas, not gas in the stomach. It can become very uncomfortable, even to the point of incapacity, at least temporarily. Though bloating can ultimately lead to belching and burping, this is usually not the case. Gas develops because of the fermentation of carbohydrates and putrefaction of proteins because of the lack of bile. True, bile has no digestive effect on carbohydrates and protein, but it does

264

have a sterilizing effect on potential fermentation and putrefactive bacteria. Therefore, when bile is lacking, these
processes can take place relatively uninhibited. This gas
forms in the small intestines and increases in amount as the
day progresses since it cannot be passed out easily. By
evening the abdominal girth may have expanded eight
inches.

GALLSTONES

Bile is produced and secreted by the liver and most of it is
stored in the gallbladder before being liberated into the
duodenum upon demand. When the flow is slow and too
much concentrating takes place in the gallbladder, sometimes stones are formed. Stones can be dissolved by increasing the flow rate and decreasing the thickness, density
and viscosity of the bile. Disodium phosphate, epsom salts,
and magnesium citrate can cause the bile to become more
liquid and flow more readily. Small dosages like ¼ to ½
teaspoonful in a glass of water at bedtime can accomplish
this in the majority of situations.

When a gallstone begins to pass through the common
bile duct, a tube from the gallbladder to the duodenum, it
sometimes becomes stuck and causes a back pressure of
bile. This causes pain known as gallbladder colic. A simple
method to cause the passing of a gallstone is to take 2
ounces each of olive oil and lemon juice at bedtime for two
nights. On the third night take 4 ounces each of the olive oil
and lemon juice. On the morning of the fourth day take a
cleansing enema followed by a coffee retention enema.
(Brew or percolate two cups of coffee using four tablespoonfuls of freshly ground regular coffee, dilute the coffee
to one pint and allow to attain room temperature. Then
inject the coffee into the rectum after cleansing enema,
using a #16 F urethral catheter, and retain the contents as

long as possible.) Your diet for these three days should be apple juice only. One gallon per day for men and 3 quarts for women.

Ordinarily the gallstones begin to pass after the third day. They pass in the stool and can be found by examining the stool. It is not unusual to pass 100 stones at one time. So long as any colic pain that may occur can be relieved by a coffee enema, there is no danger. If the enemas do not relieve pain, then it means that a stone is stuck in the neck of the gallbladder or in the common duct. This leads to surgical removal unless it becomes dislodged. However, during the combined forty years of using this technique, the authors have never seen a stone become lodged that could not be passed. Even so, if surgical removal should become necessary, it is simply that the technique brought on the inevitable sooner. The technique did not cause the stone. Actually this could be a blessing because the surgeon could remove the stone from the common duct only, and leave the gallbladder intact. If the stone were still in the gallbladder, you would probably lose the gallbladder as well.

GAS AND HALITOSIS

It may seem to the casual observer that these two symptoms are incompatible since they are involved at the opposite ends of the digestive tract. Not so, because we are dealing with the ability of the pancreas to produce the digestive capability needed to process the food consumed. When insufficient capability exists, the foods are incompletely digested: proteins are not broken down into amino acids but become putrefied; carbohydrates are not broken down into monosaccharides but become fermented; fats are not broken down into fatty acids and glycerol but become peroxidated or rancid. Among the by-products of these processes is the formation of gas. This gas is carbon dioxide and hydrogen sulphide, mostly. This accounts for the quantity as well as the aroma. These are personal as well as social problems.

While this is going on, the breakdown products of putrefaction, fermentation and rancidity are present in the intestinal tract and are absorbed into the blood. The blood circulates throughout the body, creating a degree of toxicity. This adds to the burden of detoxification or excretion by all the excretory glands like the lungs, kidneys, skin and bowels. This overload causes abnormal odors to develop in the sweat, known as body odor; and in the expired air, also known as halitosis; and in flatus or gas passed by rectum. The urine becomes very aromatic as well as the stool residue, all for the same reason — systemic toxification.

While all this is going on in the intestinal tract, the sensation of nausea is not uncommon.

The nutritional approach for this sort of problem is to improve the digestive capability of the intestinal tract, specifically the pancreas. The pancreas is involved in digestion of each of the major nutrients: protein, fat and carbohydrates. The work is done by enzymes secreted in the pancreatic juices. Certain nutrients are needed for the production of pancreatic juices, but these are the essential basic nutrients needed in general by all tissues and glands. However, by taking raw pancreatic DNA-RNA preparations, the function of the pancreas can be stimulated. One to four 450 mg. tablets of raw pancreas DNA-RNA concentrate taken before meals, stimulates the pancreas to produce more digestive juices, resulting in improvement in digestive capability. Pancreatin, an enzyme produced by the pancreas, is also of assistance. It can usually be found in a good digestive enzyme.

CROHN'S DISEASE

No doubt this condition is unknown by many. Some may remember that President Eisenhower suffered from regional enteritis. This is the same condition. It is merely an inflammation of a section of the small intestine. Symptomatically, one can say that the old-fashioned bellyache would best describe it. It is a severe and incapacitating condition and seems to be heavily overladen with allergic and emotional components.

The condition can be brought under control rather quickly by soothing the intestinal mucosa. Two simple herbal remedies can accomplish this in most situations. One is a comfrey-pepsin combination, and the other is aloe vera. Comfrey-pepsin can be taken in capsule form and the dosage can be four times daily or even hourly. There does not seem to be any toxicity involved, so the rule of thumb is to take enough to control the symptoms. The authors have never found a case that did not respond to two capsules each hour within the first several hours. This does not cure, but does control, and buys time to allow the condition to heal. Aloe vera is a very simple remedy and can be taken as frequently as needed. One can mix about four ounces of aloe vera juice into a quart of distilled water. One is to drink four glassfuls of this mixture during the daytime hours and refill the bottle with distilled water each time a drink is taken. By 6:00 p.m. one is to cease refilling the bottle but to consume the whole quart before bedtime. Repeat the process the next day. It is quite possible that a fresh mixture may be needed during the night hours for the first day or so. No problem, take as much as needed to control the symptoms. It is one of the most soothing and healing herbs known to man. Less total fluid consumed each day can be initiated as per improvement. Yes, you will have to urinate during the night for one or two nights, but this is a small price to pay for desired results.

DIARRHEA & COLITIS

Diarrhea is usually a condition of the lower bowel where the movements are of a watery nature and not formed. They are also probably increased in number per day. The condition can be the result of an acute infection as found in the "Tourista" disease, typhoid or food poisoning, or it can result from chemical irritation of the large intestine. Diarrhea can be allergic in nature or it can be mechanical. The mechanical type is where there is a lesion like cancer which tends to block the normal bowel flow which results in constipation. The stool liquifies above the lesion and passes out as diarrhea. Alternate constipation and diarrhea is a probable indication of serious problems. See your doctor immediately. Allergic irritation causes increased peristalsis hence speeded up passage through the digestive tract resulting in fluid type stools.

The irritation of the large intestine mucosa or colitis causes excessive mucus and can be very severe, even to the extent that the tissues seep bloody fluid or actually bleed. This is called bloody colitis. When the irritation continues for a prolonged period of time, the tissues of the intestinal wall tend to weaken and small outpocketings may develop. This is called diverticulosis. When the pouches become inflamed, they are called diverticulitis.

Nutritional treatment for diarrhea varies somewhat depending upon the cause. However, provision of adequate bulk in the stool is very important. Bulk or fiber absorbs some of the available water, swells up and causes the stool to become semi-solid before being passed. However, diarrhea is commonly a problem requiring more immediate action and bulk does not solve the problem. There should be an immediate cessation of eating. In very extreme situations, even water may be denied, and the patient must be fed by intravenous methods. However, water fasting is usually sufficient. The usage of comfrey-pepsin and aloe vera, as mentioned before, can be used in this condition. Montmorillonite clay or Kaopectate® can be used, two tablespoonfuls four times daily.

ELECTROLYTE LOSS

One of the dangers of continued diarrhea is the loss of electrolytes. In general, electrolytes are the mineral substances that are dissolved in the fluids of the body. Electrolyte balance is very important for health. Disturbances can be fatal in a short period of time, particularly in infants. Since there may be an inability to hold mineralized water in the gut long enough for absorption, other measures can be used to restore the electrolyte balance. Fluid and electrolytes can be put into the body via the skin. Apple cider vinegar body rubs can be put into the body via the skin. Apple cider vinegar body rubs are of great assistance because of the potassium and mineral content. Rubbing sea water into the skin adds a variety of minerals.

CONSTIPATION

Constipation is very important in our society. There are many persons who believe that one or two bowel movements a week are normal. Here is a very obvious reason why this is not true: As mentioned before, when the digestive tract does not completely digest all foods into appropriate breakdown products, the residuals undergo putrefaction, fermentation and rancidity. These toxic products cause the formation of several other chemicals which are very toxic to the system. They are present in the large bowel in all cases since the body never completely digests all food substances. The longer these products remain in the intestinal tract, the more toxic materials are absorbed into the blood. It is very simple. The longer the waste products remain in the large intestine, the more toxic chemical by-products are absorbed, resulting in more toxicity in the system. Toxicity in the system leads to all sorts of degenerative conditions depending upon the biochemical individuality of the person involved. Actually, one or two movement each day is much more normal.

The answer to this problem is quite simple in itself: give the bowel enough fiber and the accumulation of stool cannot take place. Fiber absorbs fluid, making increased amount of softer stool. The increased mass demands evacuation, thus no more constipation. It is possible that one may need an herbal laxative at first to ensure daily or oftener bowel movements. Laxatives may be phased out as the bowel becomes awakened and begins to function more normally.

SPASTIC COLITIS

A condition that may develop when there is a lack of bulk is called spastic colitis. This means that the bowel is tight or tense because the peristalsis (muscular action of the walls of the colon) is working on next to nothing inside the bowel. Since it is muscularly tight or squeezed down, it means that blood is not being circulated to the bowel wall in a normal manner. This results in hypoxia or reduced oxygen availability to the bowel wall, which causes the tissues to become acidotic from nonremoved metabolic waste products, which results in swelling of the local tissues. All this adds up to a very irrigated large intestine. It can all be solved by use of fiber along with comfrey-pepsin and aloe vera in amounts similar to that previously described.

GENERALITIES

Regarding the Use of Sugar and Protein and/or Fat Combinations — One of the little known deleterious effects of refined sugar is its reaction in the gastrointestinal tract with protein and/or fat combinations. First of all, let us establish that concentrated carbohydrates (sugars) stay in the stomach for only a short period of time since very little digestion is necessary. On the other hand, protein remains in the stomach for extended periods of time (up to 5 hours) because much activity must take place before the proteins can be passed on to the small intestine for absorption. Some fats also are broken down in the stomach and the presence of fat in the stomach slows down the production of hydrochloric acid which further delays the time of departure of stomach contents. When concentrated carbohydrates are mixed with protein or protein/fat combinations, the sugars tend to ferment in the stomach producing gas. Adequate hydrochloric acid will prevent this to some extent, but the major cause of stomach gas is improper combining of food groups. Too many Americans are accustomed to finishing off a good protein meal with sweet desserts. For best nutrition, concentrated sweets should be eaten on an empty stomach — this includes fruits, fruit juices, et cetera.

There are many sugar-protein combinations which may be easily avoided if one is on the alert; an outstanding example is eggs with orange juice. The fact that many foods contain a combination of protein and carbohydrate must be taken into consideration — such natural combinations rarely give much trouble as it is concentration of carbohydrate which produces the deleterious effects, these being proportional to the quantity present.

Allergies are involved two ways in the intestinal tract. The primary allergic tissue reaction is one of swelling and congestion of the cells involved. The gastro-intestinal tract is no different than any other tissue in this regard. The mucosa becomes swollen and congested when reacting allergically. The reaction can occur in any part of the tract from the mouth and lips all the way to the anus. Depending upon the area involved, the symptoms develop accordingly. In general, one of the most soothing elements for allergic reactions in the tract is aloe vera. Directions for use are already provided in other sections of this chapter.

The second type of allergic involvement of the intestinal tract is that when the tissues are reacting allergically, they lose their natural selective absorption powers. That is, the swollen and congested mucosal tissues lose their ability to be selective in the substances that they allow to penetrate. Case in point are the protein derivatives. Normally amino acids or basic units of proteins are usually absorbed in toto through the intestinal mucosa. When these tissues are allergically affected, some protein derivatives of compounded amino acids can be absorbed before they are broken down into amino acids. These more complex amino acid structures in themselves create more allergic reactions. It becomes a vicious circle, the more allergic reaction taking place, the more allergic tissue response develops.

One of the primary functions of vitamin A in the system is to maintain the integrity of skin and mucosal tissues. Mucosa is the "inside skin" of the intestinal tract. Remember, the intestinal tract is a tube of the outside world passing through us. Integrity of the intestinal mucosa is quite important to the individual since this area is the contact point between the outside and inside worlds.

Vitamin B complex is another group of vitamins that have special affinity for skin and mucosa. Not only does the B complex have much influence on normal intracellular metabolism for all cells in the body, it has special affinity for the ectodermal, skin and mucosa, structures. The cardinal signs of B complex deficiency are dermatitis, diarrhea, dementia (brain is also an ectodermal structure) and death.

Detoxified garlic preparations are definitely soothing to the intestinal mucosa. They have an antibiotic effect without the drawbacks of iatrogenic or doctor-induced illnesses. They are also an antiparasitic (worm) substance or vermifuge. Parasites are much more common in the human intestinal tract than is generally believed. One should always consider that parasites may be present until proven otherwise. Every person with a gastrointestinal tract complaint should be treated with detoxified garlic, enzymes and other vermifuges routinely along with all other forms of treatment.

Enzymes are a necessity for digestion. Not only that, but excesses are absorbed into the system for general beneficial effect. This is important in relation to protein digestive enzymes like trypsin and chymotrypsin (found in pancreatin), since the excesses of these enzymes are absorbed into the system to control tophoblastic or embryonic cell development, a non-differentiated precancerous-type cell. Adequacy of these enzymes keeps precancerous cells from developing.

One cannot overstress the importance of good teeth. Poor teeth and missing teeth certainly point to poor nutritional status of the person. Poor-fitting dentures and lack of hydrochloric acid seem to go together. Absence of hydrochloric acid is one factor which is almost always found along with cancer. Maintain your hydrochloric acid capacity if at all possible.

Cancer can occur at any place along the digestive tract. If the principles mentioned beforehand are followed preventively, the development of cancer is less likely than if the principles are not followed. Cancer in specific areas must be considered on the basis of the area involved, and the type of degeneration present. Please refer to our chapter on Cancer.

CONCLUSION

The digestive tract is a very active area of the body. it needs to be maintained in good operating condition at all times or else disease and disturbances develop. Usually the answers to particular problems are relatively simple to follow. Be alert and aware as to when your digestive tract is sending out body language reports that all is not well. Solve the little problems before they become complicated. It can be done.

APPENDIX

SUGGESTED DIGESTIVE ENZYME FORMULA:

Betaine HCl	120 mg.
Pancreatin	150 mg.
Bile Extract	120 mg.
Pepsin	65 mg.
Lipase	100 mg.
Papain	100 mg.

SUGGESTED VERMIFUGE PROGRAM:

1. Take a cleansing enema every other evening at bed-time for one month.

2. Apply carbolated vaseline to anal area each bedtime for one month.
3. Take a systemic enzyme preparation hourly while on a 24-hour water fast. A juice fast may be used, but this is less effective than a water fast.
4. Follow through with detoxified garlic twice or three times daily for at least a month. Detoxified garlic is a good prophylactic so should be a routine in your life.
5. Starting the day with 2 tablespoonfuls of apple cider vinegar in water is an excellent prophylaxis for many conditions.

HERBAL TIPS:

GASTROINTESTINAL — Ulcers, gastritis, heartburn, indigestion, colitis, diverticulitis.

Comfrey Leaf	Cayenne Pepper
Myrrh Gum	Peppermint

VERMIFUGE

Garlic	Mandrake
Black Walnut Leaves	Quassia

SIMPLE DIGESTANT
Apple Cider Vinegar — 1-2 tsp. in water aids digestion.

Chapter 18

NATURAL SUBSTITUTES
FOR
COMMON DRUGS

DRUGS — THEIR ACTIONS AND REACTIONS

- Does the "extra ingredient" make Anacin worth asking for?
- Should you give your cold to Contac?
- Will you sleep better tonight if you've taken Sominex?
- Can you say good-bye to a stopped-up nose if you squirt Sine-Off according to the instructions on the box?
- Does the $1.50 aspirin get into the bloodstream and bring relief more quickly than the 38 cent aspirin?
- Can tonight's Alka-Seltzer prevent tomorrow's hangover?

Let's take a look at the answers to the above questions.
- The extra ingredient in Anacin is caffeine. If that is what you want, drink a cup of coffee.
- If you want to give your cold to Contac, it might be wise to check and see if you have glaucoma, because your eyes could be irreparably damaged if you took Contac. Also one of the ingredients in Contac could cause trouble for anyone who has hypertension.

277

- Tests have indicated that Sominex is not more effective in promoting sleep than a placebo containing no medication.
- Sine-Off says to use it twice within 10 minutes and repeat every three hours. Such usage would result in rebound congestion worse than what you started with.
- The rate of dissolution of any aspirin tablet in the stomach is so nearly identical that such claims are questionable. Incidentally, don't use aspirin after you have been drinking, because alcohol changes the integrity of the cells in the stomach lining, and you will lose a certain amount of blood from the irritant in the aspirin.
- The best way to prevent a hangover is not to consume alcohol; the use of an Alka-Seltzer the night before will do nothing to prevent one.

What are you trying to tell me? That drugs don't work? No, not necessarily. Drugs certainly have their actions on the human body, but they also have reactions which can be dangerous to you. Since the theory of allopathic medicine teaches that medicine or drug is potentially curing in nature, doctors are willing to overlook the side-effects and hope for a cure. For those of you who want to follow that premise, this booklet is written to inform you of the proper use and possible side-effects of common drugs.

I have also catalogued commonly used drugs by their application and included a section at the end of each grouping on a nutritional adjunct program. This is not to be considered as a substitute for the use of these drugs, but merely information on various nutrients which might have a similar or synergistic effect. The use of drugs should be regulated by someone who is familiar with their functions and the amount of dependence that the body may achieve. Abrupt withdrawal can lead to serious complications which can be avoided with the use of common sense.

HIGH BLOOD PRESSURE DRUGS

ALDACTAZIDE — Used for treatment of high blood pressure, water accumulation due to congestive heart failure, cirrhosis of the liver, kidney disease and water retention of unknown causes. This preparation is a combination of two drugs which help the kidneys to pass water and salt and help reduce the symptoms of the above-mentioned condition.

Side-Effects: Dryness of mouth, thirst, drowsiness, tiredness, mental confusion, diarrhea, intestinal cramps, development of breasts in males, loss of sexual drive, masculinizing traits in females (including beard growth, deepening of voice and menstrual irregularities), headache, skin eruptions, hives, fever, loss of balance, abnormal bruising, loss of appetite, nausea, vomiting, rash, itching, abnormal skin sensation (including tingling, crawling and burning), yellowing of skin, yellow appearance of objects (yellow vision), increased reactivity to sunlight, muscle spasms, weakness and restlessness, sore throat, sores in the mouth.

ALDOMET — Used for lowering blood pressure in patients with sustained moderate to severe high blood pressure — not recommended for mild causes of high blood pressure.

Side-Effects: Although side effects are not as common with this drug as many others, they include slowing of the heart, nasal congestion, dryness of the mouth, constipation, gas, diarrhea, nausea, vomiting, sore tongue, blackening of tongue, swollen glands in neck, weight gain, water retention, breast enlargement, lactation, impotence, loss of sexual drive, skin rash, pain in joints and muscles, skin discomfort, shaking or tremors, nightmares, mental depression.

DIURIL — Prescribed as an agent which helps the body pass water and salt in patients who retain water due to a variety of reasons. It is also prescribed for the reduction of blood pressure in patients with high blood pressure.

Warning: Mothers should not nurse while taking this drug.

Side-Effects: Dryness of mouth, thirst, weakness, lethargy, drowsiness, restlessness, muscle pains or cramps, muscle fatigue, low blood pressure, rapid heartbeat, nausea, vomiting, loss of appetite, diarrhea, constipation, yellowing of skin or eyes, gastrointestinal distress, dizziness, numbness, headache, yellow appearance of objects, anemia, rash, hives, increased sensitivity to sunlight, fever, respiratory distress, blurred vision.

DYAZIDE — Prescribed to help pass water and salt in patients who retain abnormal amounts of water due to a variety of diseases. It is also prescribed for treatment of mild to moderate high blood pressure.

Warning: Dyazide is a potent drug. Any abnormal effects should be reported to your physician immediately.

Side-Effects: Muscle cramps, weakness, dizziness, headache, dry mouth, fainting, rash, hives, increased sensitivity to sunlight, nausea, vomiting, diarrhea, constipation, numbness, yellow vision.

HYDRODIURIL — See DIURIL

LASIX — A potent drug which helps the body to pass excessive water and salt, causing a prompt and copious flow of urine. It is used in treatment of heart diease, liver problems, kidney disease and high blood pressure. It is used where weaker agents are not deemed effective.

Warning: Lasix is not recommended for pregnant women nor for children, Lasix should be taken only under the close supervision of your physician.

Side-Effects: Abdominal pain or distension, nausea,

vomiting, weakness, fatigue, dizziness, lethargy, leg cramps, loss of appetite, mental confusion, hives, itching, skin reactions, numbness, tingling of skin, blurring of vision, diarrhea, anemia, ringing in the ears, deafness, sweet taste, oral or gastric burning, swelling headache, yellowing of skin or eyes, blood clots, thirst, increased perspiration.

REGROTON — This is a combination of drugs prescribed for the control of high blood pressure.
Warning: Regroton is a potent drug which should be used only under close supervision by your physician.
Side-Effects: Loss of appetite, gastric irritation, nausea, vomiting, diarrhea, constipation, nasal congestion, muscle cramps, dizziness, weakness, headache, drowsiness, mental depression, skin rashes, hives, anemia, restlessness, visual defects, impotence, painful urination, increased sensitivity to sunlight, yellowing of skin, yellow appearance of objects, slowing of heart, itching, skin eruptions, loss of appetite.

RESERPINE — Prescribed to control mild forms of high blood pressure.
Warning: This drug can produce severe depression in susceptible individuals. Discontinue drug at first sign of despondency, loss of appetite, early morning insomnia, impotence or self deprecation. Patients should inform an anesthesiologist of current or prior use of Reserpine if contemplating surgery.
Side-Effects: Oversecretion of stomach acid, nausea, vomiting, loss of appetite, diarrhea, heart pain, heart flutters, slowing of heartbeat, drowsiness, depression, nervousness, anxiety, nightmares, tremors, dullness of feeling, deafness, eye problems, nasal congestion, itching, rash, dryness of mouth, headache, dizziness, fainting, impotence, decreased sex drive, painful urination, muscular

aches, weight gain, breast enlargement, lactation, development of breasts in males.

SER-AP-ES — Prescribed for the control of high blood pressure.

Side-Effects: Oversecretion of stomach acid, nausea, vomiting, loss of appetite, diarrhea, chest pains, heart flutters, slowing of heart, drowsiness, depression, nervousness, anxiety, nightmares, tremors, dull sensations, deafness, eye disorders, nasal congestion, itching, rash, hives, skin eruptions, painful or difficult urination, muscle aches, weight gain, breast enlargement, lactation, breast development in males, increased heart rate, numbness or tingling of skin, yellow skin or eyes, hepatitis, constipation, yellow appearance of objects, increased sensitivity to sunlight, anemia, fever chills, diminished sex drive.

CONSIDERATIONS

Since any doctor practicing good allopathic medicine will begin a hypertensive patient on medication which assists or forces the body to eliminate fluids (diuretics), we perhaps should consider edema as a primary factor in hypertension. Edema or water-logging of the tissues physically narrows the diameter of the blood vessels by simple pressure, thus increases the pressure within. This action is similar to squeezing a hose, the smaller you make the internal diameter, the more pressure you have.

Some of the causes of edema are:

1. Lack of the mineral POTASSIUM
2. Inadequate PROTEIN in the diet
3. Poorly functioning KIDNEYS

Now since almost all of the diuretic drugs are potassium wasters (cause potassium to be excreted excessively) it can readily be seen that although relief can be obtained from the use of such drugs, one of the basic causes may be aggrevated (lack of Potassium). And, if one attempts to stop the drug, all the symptoms return — often times with greater intensity. It should be noted that such drugs do nothing for the individual who has need for more protein in his diet. Also, the malfunctioning kidney (if this is the problem) needs assistance to *build* itself up and *repair* itself. Diuretics do neither!

There are some herbs which have a diuretic action without the side effects of the drugs. So, for those of you who would like to approach this from an Organic Medicine or Preventive Medicine angle, consider these suggestions:

1. If the hypertension is due to a potassium depletion, increase your potassium consumption daily by 1200 mg. Reduce your sodium intake drastically — the easiest way is not to salt your foods.

2. Eliminate white flour and white sugar products and concentrate on protein foods and fresh vegetables.

3. Use an herbal diuretic containing some or all of the following herbs: Alfalfa, Buchu, Corn Silk, Juniper, Parsley, Uva Ursi.

4. Exercise daily. This has often proven very beneficial in stubborn cases.

5. Use the Liver-Kidney-Bowel Cleansing Fast outlined later in this book to clear up any back pressure from these organs.

6. Do not use alcoholic beverages, coffee, or black tea. (For a more complete resume of the facts on blood pressure, see the chapter entitled 'Blood Pressure'.)

ANTIARTHRITICS

INDOMETHACIN (INDOCIN) — A paradox in the drug

field, Indocin has been investigated by the American Rheumatism Association and failed to provide any more relief than a placebo. Yet this drug is widely prescribed by physicians, even when it is not generally considered to be a drug of choice for any condition.

Side-Effects: Gastrointestinal ulceration, including perforation and hemorrhage of the esophagus, stomach and small intestine, gastrointestinal bleeding, ileitis, nausea, vomiting, hepatitis, jaundice, aplastic anemia, hemolytic anemia, bone marrow depression, agranulocytosis, leukopenia, allergic reactions, deafness, tinnitus, psychic problems, coma, convulsions, dizziness, headaches, edema, hypertension and aggravation of diabetes.

CONTRAINDICATIONS — Not to be used by children, pregnant women, nursing mothers, the elderly, patients with a history of gastrointestinal problems, epilepsy, parkinsons disease.

PHENYLBUTAZONE
(BUTAZOLIDIN, FENILBUTAZOMA) — Since the incidence of arthritis is increasing by leaps and bounds, and there is such a need for a safer, more effective treatment than aspirin, drug manufacturers constantly seek for such a substance. It is also extremely obvious that phenylbutazone, commonly known as butazolidin is NOT such a substance regardless of how popular it may be with some physicians. The book "Pharmacological Basis of Therapeutics" by Drs. Goodman and Gilman states: "Indiscriminate use of phenylbutazone in the therapy of trivial acute or chronic musculoskeletal disorders can only be condemned." A variety of authoritative sources in the United States stress the dangers associated with this drug and warn that it may produce life threatening side effects.

Side-Effects: The AMA Drug Evaluation notes that

phenyl-butazone has extremely limited usefulness because of its potential toxicity. Treatment period should be limited to *one week*. Fever, rash, pruritis (itching), jaundice, weight increase, tarry stool, peptic ulcer with hemorrhage and/or perforation, ulcerative stomatitis, hepatitis, aplastic anemia, leukopenia, agranulocytosis, and thrombocytopenia. (These last three are blood disorders.)

PREDNISONE — Prednisone is a steroid (cortisone-like) type hormone derived from the cortex of the adrenal gland. Originally used for the treatment of adrenal insufficiency, it rapidly came into use for such conditions as arthritis, bronchial asthma, skin diseases, ulcerative colitis, cerebral edema, leukemia and shock. Unfortunately this is a very powerful drug with slow, cumulative toxic effects on *all* tissues, which may be inapparent until made manifest by a serious disorder caused by it. A particularly serious side effect is the *reactivation* of healed or latent tuberculosis. Eleanor Roosevelt died from reactivated tuberculosis after several months therapy with steroid hormones for anemia.
Side-Effects: Severe mental disturbances, peptic ulceration with bleeding and perforation, bone softening, spontaneous fractures of vertebrae, serious muscle damage, convulsions, glaucoma, vertigo, hypertension, heightened susceptibility to fungus, viral and bacterial infections, facial rounding, stimulation of preexisting diabetes, and edema.

While corticosteroids have a marked anti-inflammatory effect, notably in arthritic disease, they control the manifestations of the inflammation rather than the underlying disease process of tissue destruction and fibrosis (a changing of normal tissue into fibrous type tissue). In rheumatoid arthritis, progressive joint destruction continues despite the use of drugs such as prednisone.

Many physiologists have recommended that this type of drug be used only in life-threatening situations because of long term side effects which may be more serious than the condition being treated.

CONSIDERATIONS

The arthritic type disorder is a degenerative type disease. Drugs commonly used to relieve the discomfort associated with it do nothing to restore normalcy. Perhaps that is the reason arthritis foundations say there is no cure for arthritis. I do not agree with such reasoning. The human body is a constantly changing, constantly alive mechanism. Cells die and are replaced with new healthy cells if you but furnish the nutrients necessary to rebuild these cells. The following program may be of value to those who wish to approach arthritis from a positive, cell rebuilding aspect.

1. Use the LIVER-KIDNEY-BOWEL CLEANSING FAST, followed by the CREATIVE RESTORATION DIET — both are available from your local health food store or the Institute.

2. Exercise each and every day to capacity. This is a very individual thing and cannot be outlined; some may be able to do only isometric exercises while others may participate in rather vigorous activity.

3. A multiple food supplement high in pantothenic acid, vitamin C and vitamin B-6 is a must. Such a supplement should contain all the other vitamins and minerals in good balance. (For detailed discussion of the condition known as Arthritis, read the chapter entitled 'ARTHRITIS'.)

ANTIBIOTICS

How about these wonder drugs? Are they really as fantastic and/or necessary as they seem? Doctors are prescribing these antimicrobial agents in ever increasing numbers. It should be beyond question that antibiotics are among the most valuable pharmaceutical products available to the physician. However, the possibility of abuse is probably the real tragedy of life saving drugs.

Any doctor who prescribes an antibiotic for a cold or sore throat hasn't done his homework properly. If the particular infection you might have is viral in nature, you can take all the antibiotics in the world without help. Also certain of the antibiotics have an affinity for certain types of bacteria, so careful evaluation and selection of the right antibiotic is necessary.

AMPICILLIN (OMNIPEN, POLYCILLIN, PENBRITIN, PRINCIPEN, AMCILL) — This is a broad spectrum antibiotic of the penicillin family (although more expensive than penicillin and no more effective). We always live in the shadow of anaphylactic shock from the penicillins, so if you have any history of allergic reactions to penicillin, none of these drugs should be used. Death in as little as 90 seconds and up to 50 hours or more can occur.

Side-Effects: Nausea, diarrhea, vomiting, inflamed tongue, repiratory failure, skin rashes, anemia, hives, joint pain, fever.

CONTRAINDICATIONS: Pregnant women, young children — "Certain practices, such as the administration of Ampicillin to children less than 10 years of age is particularly hazardous, and their use for prophylaxis or for any situation lacking a clear indication is to be condemned" — these are the words of a medical review committee.

TETRACYCLINE (ACHROMYCIN) — A broad spectrum antibiotic of relatively low toxicity but some potentially serious side effects must be considered. Superinfections have occurred, and these may be life threatening.

Side-Effects: Liver damage, light sensitivity, overgrowth of non-susceptible organisms, dental staining in infants and young children, vomiting, diarrhea, nausea, rashes, blood changes, vaginitis.

CONTRAINDICATIONS: Do not use with penicillin or anti-coagulant therapy, or when patient suffers from gastritis, vaginitis, glossitis, dermatitis, hemorrhage, albuminuria, hematuria, or is in shock. Congenital malformations have been reported in newborn due to administration of tetracycline during the first months of pregnancy.

ERYTHROMYCIN (ERYTHROCIN, ILOTYCIN, ILO-SONE) This antibiotic is often used in upper and lower respiratory tract disorders but is classified as 'possibly' effective.

Side-Effects: Nausea, vomiting, abdominal cramping, rash, overgrowth of non-susceptible bacterial organisms.

CONTRAINDICATIONS: Should not be administered to patients with liver impairment.

CONSIDERATIONS

Infections are always with us and the antibiotics are certainly a boon for serious, acute situations. But problems have arisen because of the indiscriminate use of these drugs. For example, many physicians use antibiotics as prophylactic measures. A review of 340 patients who were hospitalized for a variety of problems and who had been given antibiotic therapy gave the following judgment:

Rational, desirable treatment .. 12.9%
Questionable treatment 21.5%
Irrational, undesirable treatment 65.6%

The undesirability of antibiotic therapy lies in several areas:

1. Antibiotics can have life threatening side effects.
2. Antibiotics are non-selective, they destroy good bacteria as well as bad ones.
3. Excessive or unnecessary therapy is a factor in the increasing number of resistant strains of microorganisms that do not respond to antibiotic therapy.

Using a non-drug approach to infections, we would approach infections this way:
1. 1,000 mg. vitamin C every hour on the hour. Vitamin C not only shores up our defense mechanism, it is considered one of the best viricides in the materia medica.
2. 10,000 units vitamin A every hour on the hour. This is particularly important in the case of mucous membrane infections (urinary and respiratory tracts).
3. 1,000 mg. bioflavonoids every hour on the hour.
4. 1 tablet adrenal-thymus combination nucleoprotein every hour.
5.. 1 tablet of a good multiple vitamin and mineral complex every hour.
6. Consume copious amounts of fluid, preferably water.

This schedule will usually control most beginning colds or flu within hours and a chronic or lingering problem will respond within 24-36 hours. Dosage is reduced accordingly. Some may feel that these are tedious measures, but remember that the body needs support constantly when it is fighting infection. The rather dramatic results should compensate you adequately for the effort.

TRANQUILIZERS

Six out of ten prescriptions filled last year were for the

drug called valium, which is considered a mild tranquilizer with particular anti-anxiety properties. Actually, comparatively little is known of the mechanism by which any of the tranquilizers or central nervous system depressants (the barbiturates) work.

We do know they have a definite action. Their spectacular rise to prominence in the drug and medical field probably stems from the fact that psychologists and psychiatrists have released many 'studies' which would link the mind of man to disease.

Without a doubt, such a link exists, but to say that 60% of mankind's ills can be treated by altering his moods and anxieties is carrying things too far. Added to this is the extreme danger of habituation that these drugs impose upon the users. Since the drug (tranquilizer or barbituate) does not remove or relieve the basic cause of the disease, but merely puts the patient in a state of mental lethargy where they don't care how they feel, when the body's tolerance to the drug is reached, you begin feeling bad again, and need ever increasing amounts of tranquilizers. All the while,the deterioration in the body (whatever caused you to feel bad in the beginning) continues.

As you can see, I am not at all convinced that disease begins in the mind. The mind, like every other organ of the body, requires certain nutrients to perform properly — when these are absent there is a good chance that the mind will malfunction, just like any other organ. Thus the indiscriminate prescription of tranquilizers is quackery at its greatest — it delays proper treatment by so changing mental and nervous system function that symptoms are masked which could lead a competent doctor to the cause of the problem. Anyway, now that you know how I feel about these 'mindbenders', let's take a look at some of them.

PHENOBARBITAL — One of the first sedatives of the

central nervous system, this drug is thought to work by blocking transmission of nerve impulses. Increased doses will produce a hypnotic type sleep.

Side-Effects: Drowsiness, lethargy, a sense of mental and physical sluggishness, skin rash, hives, localized swelling of eyelids, face or lips, drug fever, "Hangover" effect, dizziness, unsteadiness, nausea, vomiting, diarrhea, joint and muscle pains, most often in the neck, shoulders and arms. Hepatitis with jaundice has been reported. Anemia, manifested by weakness and fatigue, and a reduction of blood platelets, resulting in unusual bleeding or bruising has also been noted.

CONTRAINDICATIONS: The elderly (over 60 years of age) and the debilitated may experience agitation, excitement, confusion, and delirium with standard doses. Nursing mothers should not use it as it is found in mothers milk.

IMPORTANT — Alcohol can increase greatly the sedative and depressant actions of this drug on brain function. Should not be used in conjunction with antihistamines. It is ordinarily not advisable to drive a vehicle, pilot a plane, or operate machinery while using this drug because of the delay in reaction time, and some loss of coordination. It is not advisable to be exposed to severe cold while using this drug, as dangerous lowering of body temperature can occur. This drug can create both a physical and psychological dependence.

DIAZEPAM (VALIUM) — The advantage of a drug like valium over phenobarbital is that there is less sedation. It is intended for use primarily in anxiety states and nervous tension. It is thought (but not known) that the effect it has on the body is from a reduction in activity of certain parts of the brain.

Side Effects: Drowsiness, lethargy, unsteadiness in stance and gait, skin rashes, dizziness, fainting, blurred vision, double vision, slurred speech, nausea, menstrual irregularity, tremor, impairment of liver function, eye pain, glaucoma, emotional depression.

CONTRAINDICATIONS: In the elderly and debilitated, sensations of lightheadedness, confusion, weakness, impaired bladder control and constipation are frequent problems even on standard dosages. The findings of some recent studies suggest a possible association between the use of this drug during early pregnancy and the occurrence of birth defects, such as cleft lip. It is advisable to avoid this drug completely during the first three months of pregnancy. Even in small doses this drug is found in mothers milk and can affect the infant so it is not recommended for use by nursing mothers. Valium can produce psychological and/or physical dependence if used for an extended period of time. Extreme caution should be used when combining this drug with alcohol — the alcohol may increase the sedative effects of the valium or the valium may greatly enhance the intoxicating effects of alcohol.

CHLORDIAZEPOXIDE (LIBRIUM) — Librium is another anti-anxiety type tranquilizer very commonly prescribed. Its action is similar to valium except that the response to the intake of the drug is almost twice as long. Valium is effective within 1 to 2 hours, librium takes from 2 to 4 hours.

Side-Effects: Drowsiness, lethargy, unsteadiness in stance and gait, skin rashes, dizziness, fainting, blurred vision, double vision, slurred speech, nausea, menstrual irregularity, vivid dreaming, jaundice, impaired resistance to infections, unusual bleeding and bruising, tremors, depression, birth defects, weakness.

CONTRAINDICATIONS: Identical to Valium.

MEPROBAMATE (EQUANIL, MILTOWN) — This was one of the first transquilizers, being introduced in 1955.

Librium came along in 1960 and Valium in 1963.

Side-Effects: Similar to Librium and Valium, but with the added possibility of allergic reactions, which may produce asthmatic breathing. Also reduced urine formation, heart palpitations and sudden drop in blood pressure are factors not common to the other two tranquilizers.

CONTRAINDICATIONS: Similar to Librium and Valium.

TRIFLUOPERAZINE (STELAZINE) — This is one of the strongest of the tranquilizers with anti-psychotic properties. It is often used in mental institutions to maintain mental tranquility among patients.

Side-Effects: Drowsiness, blurring of vision, nasal congestion, dryness of mouth, constipation, impaired urination, skin rashes, hives, low-grade fever, dizziness, fatigue, weakness, insomnia, restlessness, menstrual irregularity, breast congestion, milk formation, tremors, spasms of the face, neck, back, and extremities, rolling of the eyes, grimacing, clamping of the jaw, protrusion of the tongue, difficulty in swallowing, arching of the back, cramping of the hands and feet, light sensitivity, may impair the regulation of body temperature and increase the risk of heat stroke. Obviously loaded with side effects, stelazine is however not known to be addicting as the other tranquilizers are.

CONTRAINDICATIONS: Similar to all other tranquilizers.

CONSIDERATIONS

With the plethora of side effects that are present with the use of all tranquilizers, other means should be the method of choice wherever possible. For years, the nutritionists have said that the B-Complex group of vitamins were nature's relaxants. Others have pointed to calcium and magnesium as the 'lullaby minerals', or to potassium as the muscle 'calmer'. Recently a medical 'breakthrough' occurred when a physician reported that he had taken all of his patients off anti-depressants by merely adding vitamin B-1 in large dosages to each meal.

Such knowledge and results have been the favorite of the preventive medicine physician for years, but the general concensus of opinion has been that a more well rounded approach needs to be used. Fragmented nutrition is frought with the possibilities of inducing other deficiencies because nutrients work together; there is no 'magic bullet' such as orthodox medicine seems to look for.

Thus the following program is broad in concept, but specific in those nutrients known to be deficient in the anxiety state.

1. A broad spectrum vitamin-mineral supplement containing a minimum of 50 mg. each of the B-Complex vitamins.
2. A total of no less than 1250 mg. of Calcium daily.
3. A total of no less than 500 mg. of Magnesium daily.
4. A total of no less than 1200 mg. of Potassium daily.
5. Many herbalists use such herbs as valerian, lady slipper, lobelia, scullcap, hops flowers, chamomile and mistletoe as nerve relaxants with excellent results. Such herbs either in tea or tablet form are available from your local health food stores.
6. The adherance to a diet such as the Creative Restoration Diet outlined at the end of this book.

CONCLUSION

And so we come to the end of our space. Many other drugs could be discussed, in particular the over-the-counter medications which are causing much concern and some confusion. For now, I consider it adequate to say that I firmly believe the less medication one puts into his body, the better. All of these drugs are toxic and must be reacted to by the body. If natural means are available as an alternate, they should be tried first. Health comes from building, not from destruction. Oliver Wendell Holmes once said, "I firmly believe that if all the drugs could be sunk to the bottom of the sea, it would be all the better for mankind, and all the worse for the fishes."

Chapter 19

VITAMINS

"We live in a country where we have more good doctors, more great medical schools, and more hospitals, more education, and more great scientists, and more money than any other place on earth. We hear so much about the great scientific advances that have been made in public health and medicine. And it is true that great advances have been made in certain branches of medicine. But despite all this, everybody in the country is sick. I do not know anyone anywhere who does not have some physical disability. It is hard to find a child in school any more without dental caries. Last year we had more cancer than ever before. We had more heart disease. It is the leading cause of death, killing young people before the age of forty all over the land. We had more high blood pressure, more stomach ulcers, more rheumatism, more diabetes and more mental disease. Fifty per cent of the hospital beds in America are filled with mental patients. They are running out the top windows all over the land and more mental hospitals are being built every day. Perhaps we are not so smart after all. Maybe something is wrong here. There are places in the world where these degenerative diseases do not occur. The first great fundamental reason why all of us are sick is a lack of proper nutrition." These words were spoken in 1960 by Dr. Joe D. Nichols, M.D. and are just as true today as they were then.

Since that time, we have had a great awareness of nutrition sweeping this nation, but for some reason, our health professionals have been the last to take up the torch. This chapter will be the beginning of a series on vitamins, minerals, enzymes, and proteins. Specifically, this chapter will deal with vitamins, those organic food substances found in living plant and animal matter. They are essential for growth and reproduction; the formation of antibodies, coagulation of the blood; resistance to infection; formation of intercellular substances and integrity of bones, teeth, skin, blood and nervous tissue.

Man has struggled with a demarcation between health and disease. In the same light, there has been an ongoing struggle between orthodox medicine who wishes to classify disease by the germ or virus associated with it and the nutritionist who holds that disease is merely an end result of a state of malnutrition and the germs, microbes, bacteria, and viruses can and do only exist in an environment which is not in a state of perfect health. We have ample evidence that individuals are exposed to a virus, germ, or whatever, and have no health problems therefrom. Throat cultures of random individuals indicate a high presence of the pneumococcus, a bacteria associated with pneumonia, yet none of these individuals had active pneumonia or came down with it.

What I am trying to say here is that disease does not exist in the well nourished body. Vitamins are one of the important nutrients necessary for vital function to proceed normally in the body. Clinicians wait until the disease has appreared which is associated with a vitamin deficiency before the diagnosis is made of such a deficiency. I am of the opinion that it is like closing the barn door after the horse got out. Awareness of early signs of vitamin deficiency, the total integration of all vitamins, and how to properly use vitamins as a supplement to daily food intake is what this chapter will be all about. I would like to caution you that all bodies do not function exactly the same. We are not poured out of the same mold, therefore we have peculiarities in function and reaction.

How many times have I heard the statement, "I can't take vitamin so and so, it makes me sick to my stomach, or gives me diarrhea, or gives me a headache, or gives me a rash." I never question such a reaction, because I know that the person is telling the truth. Such a statement will often give me a clue as to a malfunctioning digestive system, plugged up or missing gall bladder, or even a serious deficiency of another vitamin.. Others will have a particular need for a single vitamin because their body is not able to properly metabolize that vitamin and an extra abundance is needed to furnish minimal amounts of normal function. Niacin, also known as vitamin B-3, is an excellent example of this. Many physicians have now accepted that many, (if not all) schizophrenics have a chemical problem handling this vitamin and thus need super amounts of it. Thus, the daily needs of an individual cannot be arbitrarily set by some august body which meets once every five years. In the final determination, each individual must come to a decision at which level of nutritional support they feel best and function best. I have found personally over the years that I need more vitamin A, magnesium, potassium, and vitamin B-6 than what I would consider a good balanced supplement program. Hopefully, this chapter will assist you in finding that same level for yourself and give you that exuberant feeling where you want to tell everyone how good you feel.

THE FAT SOLUBLE VITAMINS

The fat soluble vitamins, as the term implies, are those

four vitamins (A, D, E, K) which are found in nature generally associated with fatty foods such as butter, cream, vegetable oils, and the fats of meat and fish. The general characteristics of the fat-soluble vitamins are:

1. They are more stable to heat than the water soluble vitamins and are less likely to be lost in the cooking and processing of foods.

2. Fat-soluble vitamins are absorbed from the intestine along with fats and lipids in foods, so that anything that interferes with fat absorption results in lower utilization of this class of vitamins. (Examples: The use of mineral oil seriously hampers the absorption of *any* fats; the lack of adequate bile also impairs absorption.)

3. Because these vitamins are not soluble in water, they are not excreted in the urine. Instead, they are stored in the body, chiefly in the liver.

VITAMIN A

Vitamin A is possibly the most underrated and feared of the group. On the other hand, some nutritionists feel that it is the most important of all vitamins. It is only found in the animal kingdom, but man can convert pro-vitamin A (carotene) from plant sources into vitamin A. This conversion takes place primarily in the intestinal wall during absorption and in the liver.

Functions:

1. One of the chief functions of vitamin A is to maintain the health of epithelial tissues — namely the skin and membranes that line all passages which open to the exterior of the body, as well as glands and their ducts.

2. Proper formation and maintenance of tooth enamel and health of gums.

3. Proper growth of bones.

4. Proper health of sex glands and uterus.

5. Allows night vision.

Deficiency Symptoms:

1. Predisposition to colds, infections of the respiratory and urinary tract, sinusitis, abscesses in ears and mouth, general infections.

2. Lack of ability to see well in dim light.

3. Acne.

4. Rough, dry, scaly skin.

5. Sensitivity to light.

6. Xeropthalmia (lack of tears, eyelid swollen and pus laden)

7. Reproductive difficulties (poor fertilization, abnormal embryonic growth, abortion).

FOOD SOURCES OF VITAMIN A

100 gm. Beef Liver	43,900 IU
100 gm. Carrots	11,000 IU
100 gm. Apricots, dried	10,900 IU
100 gm. Sweet Potatoes	8,800 IU
100 gm. Collards	7,800 IU
100 gm. Dandelion greens	11,700 IU
100 gm. Swiss chard	5,400 IU
100 gm. Spinach	8,100 IU
100 gm. Pumpkin	6,400 IU
100 gm. Liverwurst	6,350 IU
100 gm. Papaya	1,750 IU
100 gm. Persimmon	2,700 IU
100 gm. Cantaloupe	3,400 IU
100 gm. Nectarine	1,480 IU
100 gm. Swordfish	2,100 IU
100 gm. Oat flakes	5,000 IU
100 gm. Raisin Bran	4,675 IU

100 gm. Butter	3,300 IU
100 gm. Cheddar Cheese	1,300 IU
100 gm. Eggs, whole	1,180 IU

Note: 100 grams is equal to about three and one-half ounces.

The above have been listed in some detail because of the difficulty in readily obtaining potent amounts of vitamin A in supplementation. Where a Vitamin A deficient patient is observed, they should be encouraged to eat the above foods in addition to the supplementation.

VITAMIN K

This vitamin is the well known "coagulating factor." It is found in some foods such as alfalfa, casein, soybean oil, most green leafy vegetables and can be synthesized in the intestinal tract by the bacterial flora. It is considered good preventive medicine to administer Vitamin K to the pregnant mother to prevent hemorrhaging and also to prevent the possibility of hypoprothrombinemia in the infant. Very little is stored in the body, but what is stored is in the liver.

Function of Vitamin K:
Formation of prothrombin in the liver.

Deficiency Symptoms:
1. Delayed blood clotting.
2. Internal bleeding.
3. Subcutaneous hemorrhage.

It should be noted that individuals who have been on antibiotic therapy with a resultant decrease or loss of intestinal flora often suffer from a deficiency of vitamin K because the body depends on a daily synthesis of this vitamin in the intestinal tract. It has therefore been suggested that the use of acidophilus liquid or capsules concommitantly and after such antibiotic therapy makes good sense.

VITAMIN D

This vitamin is often overlooked because we think that all that is necessary is exposure to sunlight. In effect, that is true, but so many now live in congested areas where fog, smog and other pollutants prevent the ultraviolet spectrum of the sun from reaching our exposed skin where a derivative of cholesterol (7-dehydrocholesterol) is converted by the ultraviolet of cholecalciferol (vitamin D-3). In plant life, a substance known as ergosterol is converted to ergocalciferol which is classified as vitamin D-2. Vitamin D belongs to a class of organic substances known as STEROLS which are the precursors in the body of many important hormones.

Functions of Vitamin D:

1. Promote growth and proper mineralization of the bones and teeth. This is accompanied by the proper utilization of calcium and phosphorus.

2. Formation of specific forms of ribonucleic acid.

3. Formation of specific enzymes.

Deficiency Symptoms:

1. Poor growth and lack of normal bone development.

2. Rickets (bowlegs, knock-knees, enlargement of bones at ends, beading of the ribs).

3. Osteomalacia (softening of bones in adults).

4. Fatigue.

5. Arthritis.

6. Defective teeth.

7. Enlarged skull.

Food Sources:

100 gm. Herring	....	330 IU
100 gm. Salmon	....	314 IU
100 gm. Tuna	....	260 IU

VITAMIN E

Although we are often criticized for associating vitamin E with the reproductive organs and functions in the body, this particular vitamin was discovered because of animals' inability to reproduce on a Vitamin E deficient diet. When foods containing this substance were added to the diet, reproduction capacity was restored. Thus there is substantial basis for the supposition that vitamin E has a beneficial effect on the organs of reproduction.

Probably the most misunderstood aspect of vitamin E intake is its concomitant use with iron. *Vitamin E is absolutely essential for the adequate absorption of iron* but certain types of iron use up more of the Vitamin E than others. We will delineate proper iron preparations later, but it is not a nutritional sin to supply vitamin E with iron at the same time — providing the formula is not composed of Ferrous Sulfate or Ferrous Chloride.

Another frequently asked question refers to a degree of superiority — Is d-alpha tocopherol better than mixed tocopherols or vice versa? First of all, understand that before we knew about tocopherols of any kind, wheat germ and wheat germ oil was producing all the effects we now ascribe to vitamin E. And these products contained all the tocopherols — our only advantage now is that we can concentrate them and we know that the alpha portion is the most biologically active. Also the law now requires that all vitamin E supplements be labelled for the alpha content, so if you buy a 100 IU mixed tocopherol capsule you get 100 IU of alpha plus whatever beta, delta, gamma and zeta tocopherols the particular oil carries. I prefer wheat germ oil as the base because it is the finest source of balanced tocopherols.

Regarding water soluble vitamin E preparations, it is my opinion that the conversion of an oil soluble substance (designed so by nature) to a water soluble substance must change its activity in the body. It has been my experience that the water soluble substances do not give the results I would expect from vitamin E. Furthermore, the only reason for using water soluble vitamin E is an inability to digest oils and fats. This is a *cardinal indication* of a liver — gallbladder problem and should be dealt with from that aspect instead of trying to run around it.

Functions of Vitamin E:
1. The most important function of vitamin E is its ability to prevent peroxide formation. It does this because of its anti-oxidant properties and these are particularly important when a diet is rich in unsaturated oils.
2. Protects all the fat-soluble vitamins.
3. Protects the pituitary, adrenal and sex hormones.
4. Prevents scar tissue formation — internally and externally.
5. Increases the rate at which new blood vessels develop around damaged areas.
6. Protection against noxious agents (carbon tetrachloride, alloxan and methyl cholanthrene).
7. Assists in normalizing blood viscosity.
8. Protects against muscle degeneration.
9. Maintains normal permeability of capillaries.

Deficiency Symptoms:
1. Male — Non-motility of spermatozoa; loss of sex instinct.
2. Female — Spontaneous abortion, uterine degeneration, sterility.

3. Retarded growth in children.
4. Progressive nutritional muscular dystrophy.
5. Swelling and hyalinization of skeletal and cardiac muscle which becomes necrotic.
6. Menstrual discomfort.
7. Angina pectoris.

WATER SOLUBLE VITAMINS

The water soluble vitamins consist of the B Complex and vitamin C. They are thus named because of the ready ability to have an excess passed off in the urine rather than being stored as the fat soluble ones tend to be. They also are absorbed more completely and with less difficulty than the fat solubles because they do not rely upon adequate bile being present

VITAMIN C

Vitamin C (Ascorbic Acid) is probably the least stable of the vitamins and is very sensitive to oxygen. Its potency can be lost through exposure to light, heat, and air, which stimulate the activity of oxidative enzymes. Since so much controversy has been aroused by the large doses recommended by certain researchers, we probably know more about this vitamin than any other because of the barrage of studies done to prove or disprove the many claims made.
Functions of Vitamin C:
1. Formation and maintenance of collagen protein. (Collagen protein is tissue "cement" for skin, cartilage, tendon, and bone.)

2. Maintain strength in blood vessels.
3. Promotes sound healing of wounds.
4. Influence formation of hemoglobin, absorption of iron from intestinal tract, and deposition of iron in liver tissue.
5. Assists in the secretion of hormones from adrenals.
6. Protect the body against infections and bacterial toxins. Also against viruses.
7. Converts folic acid to folinic acid.
8. Aids in the metabolism of phenylalanine and tyrosine and tryptophan.
9. Antihistamine action.
10. Diuretic action.

Deficiency Symptoms:
1. Pink or hemorrhagic skin follicles.
2. Hemorrhages in the eye.
3. Inflammed gums.
4. Joint pains.
5. Excessive loss of hair.
6. In children — restlessness, irritability.
7. Listlessness, lack of endurance.
8. Fleeting pains in legs and joints.
9. Small hemorrhages under skin.
10. Gums which bleed easily.

COMMENT: Many feel that a group of substances which are sometimes called vitamin P (bioflavonoids, rutin, and hesperidin) are synergistic in action to vitamin C. They are often found in combination with vitamin C in nature and often the functions and deficiency symptoms are identical. It is for this reason that many manufacturers have included them in formulations although the FDA does not recognize their need in the body.

VITAMIN B COMPLEX

All B-Complex vitamins are water-soluble substances that can be cultivated from bacteria, yeasts, fungi, or molds. They are active in providing the body with energy, basically by converting carbohydrates into glucose, which the body burns to produce energy. They are necessary for normal functioning of the nervous system and may be the single most important factor for health of the nerves.

VITAMIN B-1 (THIAMINE)

Thiamine is a water soluble vitamin that combines with pyruvic acid to form a coenzyme necessary for the breakdown of carbohydrates into glucose. It is vulnerable to heat, air, and water in cooking. The best sources are the germ and bran of wheat and the hulls of rice, all of which are discarded by much of society today.

Functions of Vitamin B-1:
1. Assists in conversion of carbohydrates to glucose.
2. Stabilizes the appetite.
3. Gastrointestinal tonus.
4. Necessary for growth, fertility, lactation.
5. Necessary for normal function of nervous system.

Deficiency Symptoms:
1. Cardiac — Palpitations, gallop rhythm, enlarged heart, elevated venous pressure, myocardial lesions.
2. Polyneuritis.
3. Loss of ankle and knee jerk reflexes.
4. Toe and foot drop.
5. Muscular weakness progressing to atrophy.
6. Mental instability, forgetfulness, vague fears, feeling of persecution, confusion.
7. Fatigue.
8. Loss of appetite.

A deficiency of thiamine not only makes it difficult to digest carbohydrates but also leaves too much pyruvic acid in the blood. This causes an oxygen deficiency that produces many of the symptoms listed above.

VITAMIN B-2 (RIBOFLAVIN)

Riboflavin is a difficult vitamin to describe because it is involved in so many of the body processes. Its activity is however a "partnership" arrangement with other nutrients to form enzymes and coenzymes. It is particularly involved with the "oxidation-reduction" reactions within the tissues where hydrogen and oxygen are finally combined to form water.

Functions of Vitamin B-2:
1. Assists the eye in light adaptation.
2. Assists the conversion of tryptophan to niacin.
3. Assists in the metabolism of carbohydrates, proteins and fats.

Deficiency Symptoms:
1. Cracks and sores in corner of mouth (cheilosis).
2. Red-purple, shiny tongue (glossitis).
3. Sensation of sand on inside of eyelids.
4. Eye fatigue, burning, itching, sensitivity to light.
5. Capillary congestion of the sclera (white) of the eye.
6. Cataracts.
7. Scaling greasy dermatitis, especially in naso-labial folds and scrotum.
8. Impaired erythrocyte formation, resulting in anemia. This has just been confirmed.

VITAMIN B-3 (NIACIN or NIACINAMIDE)

The most common question regarding this B complex

vitamin is if there is a difference between niacin and niacinamide. The difference, chemically, lies in the fact that niacin contains an organic acid group and niacinamide contains an amino group. Physiologically, niacin produces vasodilation while niacinamide does not. Niacinamide produces nausea in about one percent of the people taking it supplementally and then usually only on doses of over 500 mg. at a time. Although there is some professional difference of opinion as to which is the best therapeutically, there is no clear cut evidence of one form being superior to another with the one exception of a desired vasodilatory effect in which case niacin must be used. The common form found in plant life is niacin, in animal life niacinamide is found. The amino acid tryptophan is chemically converted to niacin in the body tissues and a small amount can be synthesized by the intestinal flora. Thus a lack of protein in the diet or a lack of intestinal flora could compound a lack of niacin in the diet.

Functions of Vitamin B-3:

1. The chief function of niacin in the body is to form the active portion of coenzymes that play an essential role in tissue oxidations — thus it is necessary for the health of all tissue cells.

Deficiency Symptoms:

1. Pellagra — dermatitis, diarrhea, dementia.
2. Loss of appetite, indigestion.
3. Small ulcers, canker sores.
4. Schizophrenia.
5. Burning hands and/or feet.

VITAMIN B-6 (PYRIDOXINE)

It was welcome news indeed when the scientific community gave vitamin B-6 recognition in its RDAs. Up to that time this very important nutrient had to be labelled as an unknown quantity, even though 17 years earlier dramatic deficiencies were produced in babies fed a commercial infant food which had most of the B-6 destroyed by the heat used to sterilize the product. (Note: How many other nutrients are similarly destroyed in many of the commercial foods we consume today?)

Functions of Vitamin B-6:
1. Essential for the complete metabolism of many of the amino acids.
2. Essential for the metabolism of fats, particularly the essential unsaturated fatty acids.
3. Involved in antibody production.
4. Helps maintain sodium-potassium balance.
5. Involved in proper DNA and RNA action.
6. Facilitates glycogen conversion to glucose.

Deficiency Symptoms:
1. Dermatitis, glossitis, cheilosis.
2. Numbness of hands and feet.
3. Green tinted urine. (Xanthurenic acid)
4. Dizziness, nausea, vomiting.
5. Kidney stones.
6. Nervous disturbances including confusion and convulsions.
7. Edema.
8. Personal observation — I have often found that individuals who have low levels of B-6 or who have difficulty utilizing it, thus requiring large amounts, have either hypoglycemia or diabetes. This could be involved with the need for B-6 in converting glycogen to glucose — if not present the body demands something sweet quickly to furnish fuel. This can lead to the breakdown of the adrenals or pancreas resulting in hypoglycemia or diabetes. If diabetic, the patient usually has difficulty adjusting the insulin intake because of the erratic glycogen conversion. Remember, this is a personal observation and not substantiated.

VITAMIN B-12

This is the most complex of all the B vitamins and is the only one which has not been synthesized until early 1977 when its successful synthesis was announced. It is also unique in requiring the mineral cobalt in the center of its molecule — giving rise to the name 'cobalamin' or 'cyanocobalamin'. Neither man nor animal is able to synthesize it and even the higher forms of plant life are unable to produce it. Only the lowly fungi and bacteria manufacture vitamin B-12, although in some animals these microorganisms accomplish this process in the intestinal tract. Vitamin B-12 is dependent upon *"intrinsic factor" for its* absorption. The intrinsic factor is a mucoprotein which tightly binds with the vitamin and facilitates its absorption in a similar manner as a mineral is chelated for better absorption.

Functions of Vitamin B-12:
1. Essential for normal functioning of all cells, particularly bone marrow, nervous system, and the gastrointestinal tract.
2. Very important in formation of nucleic acids.
3. Due to its need by the bone marrow, it is needed by the body for red blood cell formation.

Deficiency Symptoms:
1. Sore tongue, weakness, loss of weight.
2. Back pains.
3. Tingling of the extremities.
4. Apathy.
5. Pernicious anemia — anemia with degeneration of the spinal cord. (Diminished reflexes and sensory perception, ataxia, stammering, jerking of limbs.)

PANTOTHENIC ACID
(D-CALCIUM PANTOTHENATE)

Function of Pantothenic Acid:

Pantothenic Acid is necessary for the makeup of *Co-enzyme A*. This factor is involved in the intermediary metabolism of carbohydrates, fats, and proteins (for their synthesis, breakdown, and release of energy). Coenzyme A is also needed for the formation of the sterols including adrenocortical hormones. It is also essential for the synthesis for acetylcholine (an important regulator of nerve tissue) and other important body compounds.

COMMENT: I think it important at this time to stress the fact that thiamin, riboflavin, biotin, niacin, pyridoxine, phosphorus, sulfur, magnesium and manganese are all involved in many of the functions listed above. The very important inter-relationship of all these nutrients coordinating for the common good of the body puts one in mind of the "All Or None" law which governs the essential amino acids. We should remember this when suggesting supplements and not allow extravagant claims for a single nutrient to lead us down the wrong path.

Deficiency Symptoms:

1. Fatigue, headache, personality changes.
2. Postural hypotension, dizziness, rapid heart rate on exertion.
3. Gastric distress, constipation (brought about by a reduction of HCl acid and pepsin secretion).
4. Numbness and tingling of hands and feet.
5. Burning sensation of hands and feet.
6. Tendency toward hypoglycemia, arthritis.

BIOTIN

The biotin naturally present in the yolk of the egg is

probably of very little value to the body when consumed as a raw egg because of the action of avidin, but the biotin needs of the body can be met with other foods. Raw eggs can offer excellent food value, particularly in the complete protein area since it has an extremely high protein efficiency ratio.

Functions of Biotin:
1. Essential in the formation of nucleic acids.
2. Essential in the formation of glycogen.
3. Required in the synthesis of several of the non-essential amino acids.

Deficiency Symptoms:
1. Dermatitis and sore tongue.
2. Loss of appetite and nausea.
3. Low-grade anemia, lassitude, insomnia.
4. Muscle pain.
5. Intense depression.

CHOLINE

Although Choline is not classified by some experts as being necessary to life, it has several catalytic and metabolic functions. It has been demonstrated to be essential for the growth of rats and it has been confirmed that it prevented the accumulation of fat in the liver in animals fed choline-low diets. Choline is the active factor in lecithin and a member of the *lipotropic* family which includes choline, betaine, methionine and inositol.

Functions of Choline:
1. Aids in metabolism of fats.
2. As a constituent of acetylcholine, it assists normal nerve function.
3. Assists in the synthesis of certain hormones such as epinephrine (adrenalin).

314

Deficiency Symptoms:
1. Fatty degeneration of liver.
2. Hemorrhagic lesions in kidneys.
3. Heart muscle lesions.
4. Atherosclerosis.

INOSITOL

Here again we have a nutrient factor that nutritionists are unable to agree upon. Since man appears capable of synthesizing this substance, it does not technically fit the definition of a vitamin, although many classify it under the B Complex group.

Functions of Inositol:
1. Aids in metabolism of fats.
2. Growth factor.

Deficiency Symptoms:
1. Atherosclerosis.
2. Exzema

FOLIC ACID (FOLACIN)

Functions of Folic Acid:
1. Necessary for synthesis of nucleic acids.
2. Necessary for synthesis of certain amino acids.
3. Prevention of macrocytic anemia.
4. Utilization of amino acids.

Deficiency Symptoms:
1. Macrocytic anemia — lack of mature red blood cells, red blood cells are larger than normal and contain less hemoglobin than normal.
2. Smooth, red tongue.
3. Gastrointestinal disturbances, diarrhea.
4. Birth deformities — cleft palate, brain damage.

COMMENT: The law prevents therapeutic amounts of

folic acid to be sold without prescription because the fatigue symptoms of pernicious anemia can be temporarily overcome by its use and allow serious nerve degeneration to take place. Rather than restricting this important vitamin, it would seem to me that the sane solution would be to require that vitamin B-12 and instrinsic factor be added to all higher potency folic acid products as this would take care of the pernicious anemia conflict.

Sources of Folic Acid:

Because of the limits this vitamin can be obtained in supplemental form, I feel that the high folic acid containing foods should be listed.

Brewers Yeast	2mg./100gm.
Liver	3mg./100gm.
Wheat Germ	.3mg./100gm.
Soy Flour	.4mg./100gm.
Garbanzo Beans	.125mg./100gm.
Various Greens .. approx.	.1mg./100gm.
Wheat Bran	.2mg./100gm.

Note: 100 grams is approximately three and one-half ounces.

PARA-AMINOBENZOIC ACID (PABA)

This food factor is also considered by some to belong to a nonessential nutrient grouping although many still classify it as a part of the whole B-Complex. High potencies are prescription items because of its neutralizing effect on the little used drug, sulfanilamide. The lesson is that many should be deprived because of a few doctors practicing antique medicine.

Functions of PABA:

1. Helps to prevent eczema and loss of pigmentation, referred to as vitiligo.
2. High amounts are effective in burn pain control.

3. Facilitates the body's production of folic acid.
4. Acts as a part of the coenzyme system.

Deficiency Symptoms:
1. Gastrointestinal disorders.
2. Fatigue, irritability, depression.
3. Pigmentation loss in skin in patches.
4. Lupus Erythematosus (doses of 16 grams daily provided a 70% response).
5. Scleroderma.

PANGAMIC ACID

Some feel that this substance, of which much is yet to be known, belongs to the B Complex — as B-15. This is common use only and not accepted as such by the FDA, but regardless of its classification, this substance is receiving much attention in other countries, especially Russia where both cardiac patients and athletes are reporting benefits from it.

Functions of PANGAMIC ACID:
1. Keeps fat from infiltrating the liver.
2. Serves as a detoxification agent.
3. Increases the body's efficiency in using oxygen.
4. Regulates blood levels of steroids.
5. Extends cell lifespan.

Deficiency Symptoms:
1. Premature aging.
2. Asthma, emphysema.
3. Cirrhosis, hepatitis, jaundice of the liver.
4. Possibly glaucoma.
5. Fatigue.
6. Heart palpitation, angina pains.

CONCLUSION

Now that you have the basic facts on the vitamins, you are probably wondering how much of each you should consume each day. I have therefore outlined my "Master Formula" for vitamin supplementation. This particular formula is hypothetical only and for illustration and it should be remembered that I *never, under any circumstance,* recommend a vitamin supplement without a mineral complement. My chapter on minerals will give you my suggestions on these nutrients.

The amounts listed here are from my experience and may not agree with certain agencies of the government and/or other so-called scientific bodies who have taken it upon themselves to limit or suggest limitations of these essential nutrients. They do reflect to the best of my knowledge, the minimal amounts needed each day for optimum health in this strained world.

Vitamin A	25,000IU
Vitamin D	1,000IU
Vitamin E	400IU
Vitamin B-1	60mg
Vitamin B-2	60mg
Vitamin B-3 (Niacin)	60mg
Vitamin B-6	60mg
Vitamin B-12	100mcg
Pantothenic Acid	120mg
PABA	60mg
Choline	60mg
Inositol	60mg
Folic Acid	400mcg
Biotin	100mcg
Vitamin C	1200mg

Now here is the plan to find your specific supplementation. Use the above vitamin pattern with the mineral pattern outlined in the chapter on minerals for 60 days. Then, if any of your complaints are still present, check the function and deficiency symptom pattern for each vitamin and mineral. Under most circumstances, your particular complaint will then be sufficiently isolated that it will be easy to find. Increase that particular nutrient gradually until you find your optimum level of intake. Common sense will soon have you on the very best nutritional support possible, designed just for you!

DEFINITIONS

POSTURAL HYPOTENSION — A phenomenon which occurs in certain individuals, usually with sluggish adrenal glands, wherein the blood pressure falls on arising from a lying position. This is most often due to delayed reaction of the adrenals which would normally send out a hormone which would tighten up the blood vessels in the body to overcome the temporary change in gravity force which would pull the blood to the lower extremities, leaving a short supply for the brain.

GLYCOGEN — The storage form of glucose, which is the form of sugar the body uses for energy. When an excess of glucose is formed from the food we consume, a part of that glucose will have a molecule of water removed chemically and be stored in the liver and muscle tissue as reserve sugar. Upon demand, such as exercise or delay of eating, this will automatically be converted to glucose to prevent energy drop.

LUPUS ERYTHEMATOSUS — A puzzling skin disorder characterized by inflammatory changes in the skin, with raised welts that can occur anywhere on the body.

SCLERODERMA — A disease of the skin characterized by hard, thickened epithelium. Has been referred to as 'elephant skin'.

Chapter 20

MINERALS

Minerals can be referred to as the 'unsung heroes of life' because they do not receive the attention that vitamins do in most literature. For one thing, minerals have always been recognized as essential to human nutrition, even long before vitamins were discovered. When vitamins were discovered about 75 years ago, they captured the imaginations of scientists and lay people alike and have pretty much held the spotlight ever since.

Another possible reason for some lag in mineral studies is the difficulty in preparing a specific mineral deficient diet. Although vitamins are used in the body in comparatively small amounts, many minerals are needed in quantities of one gram or more daily. This can also be a problem when recommending mineral supplements — often the patient must take several tablets daily in order to receive a therapeutic benefit.

I would like to point out that our need for minerals is as essential as our need for oxygen. The body can tolerate a deficiency of vitamins for a longer period of time than it can a deficiency of minerals. A slight change in the blood concentration of important minerals may rapidly endanger life. Many of the farming practices engaged in today do not encompass the restoration of balanced minerals into the soil. Thus, the vegetables, cereals, and fruits which we depend on for our supply of minerals can be seriously depleted. Reports of crops yielding only 20% of the normal iron content are not unusual.

Neither muscles nor nerves function properly unless they are bathed in tissue fluids which contain certain amounts of mineral salts. Calcium ions seem to have a stimulating effect, which tends to counterbalance the more or less relaxing effects of potassium, magnesium, and sodium. Reduced or imbalanced concentrations of these ions can result in paralysis or convulsive movements. This balance is regulated chiefly by hormones — and we must remember that these hormones rely upon certain fatty acids, vitamins, and amino acids for their manufacture. Thus, we have another important tie linking all nutrients together.

ACID — BASE BALANCE

We should consider the minerals under this heading because of the very important part they play in the regulation of the acid base balance. The cells function best in a slightly alkaline medium, and will be unable to function if the pH within the cells or in fluids surrounding the cells differs too widely from the optimum. Hence, there are elaborate mechanisms for keeping the blood and tissue fluids within a narrow pH range which falls between 7.35 and 7.45.

Mineral elements participate in regulating body neutrality in that some of them are acidic and others are basic, and these can be paired to form neutral salts. Since the preponderance of metabolic waste is in the form of some type of acid, the body often unites some of the base minerals with these waste acids and eliminates them through the urine. Other mechanisms the body has for holding its normal pH are proteins and carbonates which act as buffers (can absorb either acid or base). Very rarely is an alkalinity a problem, although overdosage of the over-the-counter stomach alkalizers has been known to produce this condition. Phosphorus, sulfur and chlorine containing foods will rapidly overcome such a condition (meats, eggs, cereals).

CHELATION

When minerals are discussed, it is essential that the subject of chelation be covered. Recently a great deal of interest has focused on chelation as a form of more efficiently absorbed minerals. Consensus of opinion is unanimous that the ability of the body to receive the mineral substance through the intestinal wall in a chelated form is the way in which Nature handles all minerals normally in the intestinal tract. The problem with stomachic chelation can be most easily demonstrated by outlining the various steps in the process:

1. Mineral is ionized — Example: Calcium lactate is split into basic calcium and carbon, hydrogen, and oxygen.
2. Protein, which *must* be present, is broken down to amino acids by hydrolyzing effect of hydrochloric acid and other digestants.
3. Free amino acids attach themselves around the bare mineral and form an easily absorbed molecule.

It is apparent that several factors must be present simultaneously in order for optimum chelation to take place in the stomach:

A. Minerals and proteins must be taken in at the same time.
B. Adequate digestive acids must be present to ionize the minerals and also break down the proteins to amino acids.
C. The amino acids must combine in a stable formation

with the base minerals — necessitating an abundance of certain amino acids.

Under ideal conditions this occurs daily but, as most of us are aware, there is an apparent breakdown of the process somewhere along the line all too often. Perhaps inadequate minerals in the diet, inadequate protein or inadequate digestive factors. Any of these can seriously hamper the normal process of chelation.

Now we come to the various methods by which external chelation can be accomplished. There are many weak chelates, including the common gluconates, citrates, and ascorbates; but I can assure you that all our research has indicated these compounds are very unstable and are ionized in the stomach, thus reverting back to a base mineral which then must be chelated by the procedure outlined above. The hydrolized protein, which is a simulation of what takes place naturally in the stomach is by far the most stable because the protein 'cover' built around the mineral is in the end stage of digestion, therefore no more breakdown occurs.

Remember that chelated minerals are absorbed up to 10 times the rate of non-chelates and you have the possibility of upsetting the balance in the body by using single mineral chelates. My experience has been that a multiple chelate is preferable.

CALCIUM

Although many books on nutrition combine the study of calcium with phosphorus, I believe that they should be considered separately because of the distinct differences in function. Calcium is the most abundant mineral in the body. It is estimated that 99 percent of the calcium in the body is deposited in the bones and teeth and the remainder is in the soft tissues. The ratio of calcium to phosphorus in the bone is 2.5 to 1. To function properly, calcium must be accompanied by *magnesium, phosphorus,* and vitamins A, C, and D.

Functions of Calcium:
1. Necessary for acid-base equilibrium.
2. Balances potassium and sodium for muscle tone.
3. Necessary for heartbeat regulation.
4. Assists in blood clotting.
5. Markedly affects muscle irritability.
6. Required for normal nerve transmission.
7. Activates several hormones necessary in metabolism.

Deficiency Symptoms:
1. Stunted growth.
2. Poor quality and malformation of bones and teeth.
3. Calcium tetany — leg cramps.
4. Excessive menstruation — lengthy menstruation.
5. Nervousness, irritability.

Calcium is rather poorly absorbed, with possibly only 30 percent or less of the ingested amount actually being taken up by the body. The factors which influence calcium absorption are: acid media in stomach, adequate amounts of vitamins A, D, and C; adequate protein and fat in the diet. Absorption takes place primarily in the duodenum and since this is only from 10 to 12 inches in length, time plays a very important role.

PHOSPHORUS

Phosphorus has more functions than any other mineral in the body. Although the body uses up phosphorus at a rate one and one-half times that of calcium, most of our diets are quite high in the phosphorus element from the protein foods (meat, fish and poultry) and the cereals. About 80 percent of the phosphorus in the body is found in the bones and teeth and about 20 percent is found in the soft tissue cells — where it is vitally concerned with normal function.

Functions of Phosphorus:
1. Formation of strong bones and teeth.
2. Acts as a blood buffer to maintain pH.
3. Essential constituent of nucleoproteins.
4. Essential fat metabolism factor — phospholipids.
5. Part of enzyme system which activates the oxidation of carbohydrates — glucose and glycogen.
6. A constituent of myelin sheath of nerves.

Deficiency Symptoms:
1. Poor bone and tooth structure.
2. Arthritis, pyorrhea, rickets.
3. Mental and physical fatigue.
4. Irregular breathing.

A calcium phosphorus balance exists in the body which is necessary for normal function. An excessive consumption of sugar seriously upsets this balance — it has been postulated that the reason the polio season was always in the summer is that the great increase of the soft drink and ice cream consumption with the concentrated sugars contained upset the calcium-phosphorus balance. Phosphorus is also absorbed rather efficiently as compared to calcium, so care should be taken that calcium intake in supplemental form be at least twice that of phosphorus in order to be balanced.

POTASSIUM

Potassium is found mostly in the cells as compared to sodium which is found in extracellular fluids. Although greatly ignored by many, the need for potassium intake is approximately 2500 mg., more than twice that of calcium or phosphorus. The probable reason for the lack of emphasis on this important mineral is the fact that it is widely distributed in many of our common foods and the daily requirement is not difficult to achieve. The use of diuretics, cortisones or conditions like diarrhea, vomiting, severe trauma, diabetes, renal disease, and excessive salt intake can all lead to a negative potassium balance in the body.

Functions of Potassium:
1. Stimulates nerve impulses for muscle contraction.
2. Acts with Sodium to regulate fluids.
3. Helps maintain slight alkaline pH of internal fluids.
4. Acts as a stimulant to the kidneys.
5. Assists in conversion of glucose to glycogen.
6. Necessary for normal health of adrenals.

Deficiency Symptoms:
1. Edema.
2. Muscular weakness.
3. Tachycardia and/or irregular heartbeat.
4. Nervousness.

One way to help the normal balance of sodium and potassium is always to use a salt which is a mixture of potassium and sodium chloride. This salt does not have the bitter taste which is objectionable to so many that straight potassium chloride exhibits. It is also readily available at most grocery and drug stores as well as health food stores.

Although governmental agencies have seen fit to limit the amount of potassium in one tablet to 99 mg., many with severe deficiencies have taken 5,000 mg. daily with nothing but good results. The average use is about 1,000 mg. daily as a supplement.

SODIUM

Practically all the sodium in the body is found in the

extracellular fluid. Probably the major function of sodium is working with chlorine to regulate the pH of the body fluids. This works by a mechanism of the kidneys whereby chlorine is excreted if the tendency is toward the acid side and sodium is excreted if the tendency is toward the alaline.

Functions of Sodium:
1. Regulates the internal fluid pH.
2. With potassium, regulates the body fluids.

Deficiency Symptoms:
1. Dehydration.

Excessive Intake Symptoms:
1. Edema.
2. Hypertension, often associated with renal damage.

We often take in sodium in ways that we are not aware — a good example being that of artifically softened water. This process adds two parts of sodium for every part of calcium or magnesium removed from the water. I heartlly suggest that you *do not drink softened water*. Also, I highly recommend that your salt supply for seasoning be a combination of sodium and potassium chloride which is readily available. It is noteworthy that *adrenal cortex insufficiency creates a desire for salt* because a regulatory hormone (aldosterone) controlling the sodium retention in the body is deficient.

CHLORINE

Although a rarely discussed mineral, chlorine is nevertheless an essential nutrient in man. It is very rarely deficient, since we consume chlorinated water plus the seasoning salts (sodium and potassium) are in the form of chlorides which yield about 60 percent chloride per volume. The major function of Chlorine is as a part of Hydrochloric Acid.

MAGNESIUM

Magnesium has only recently been allocated the importance due it as an important mineral nutrient in the body. It is rather poorly absorbed, with less than 35 percent of the ingested amount being absorbed. The recommended daily allowance is from 400 to 450 mg. so you must take in over 1200 mg. daily just to assure yourself of this minimal amount.

Functions of Magnesium:
1. Activator of many enzyme systems.
2. Essential for maintenance of DNA and RNA.
3. Necessary for normal contraction of muscles.
4. Necessary for synthesis of certain amino acids.

Deficiency Symptoms:
1. Excessive irritability of nerves and muscles.
2. Nervous tics and twitches (B-6 also involved).
3. Irregular heart beat.
4. Convulsions and seizures.

The heart beat is begun when the nerve impulse reaches the very thin filament on the heart muscle cell known as actin. Calcium provides the stimulus for the actin to reach with a magneticlike action toward the center of the cell, thus creating a contraction. Magnesium then comes into play by repelling the calcium and relaxing the muscle cell. Both magnesium and calcium are often found in short supply in cardiac problems. They share many functions and should always be used together in a ratio of approximately 2 parts calcium to 1 part magnesium.

IRON

It is estimated that 25 percent of the population in the United States is deficient in this mineral. This fact is perplexing to some because iron is a rather common mineral plus it is very inexpensive as a supplement. What is probably not taken into consideration is that only 10 percent of the ingested amount is usually absorbed. Also an adequate amount of hydrochloric acid in the stomach is imperative, plus vitamin C, vitamin E, and a protein called gastroferrin. Gastroferrin seems to regulate the absorption through the mucosal cells.

Functions of Iron:
1. Small amounts of iron are found in every tissue cell and in the components of each cell — the cell nucleus, the protoplasm, and the enzymes. These iron containing substances are largely responsible for the uptake of oxygen by the cells and in the use of oxygen in their life processes.
2. A part of hemoglobin which carries oxygen.

Deficiency Symptoms.
1. Anemia — pale skin, abnormal fatigue.
2. Shortness of breath.
3. Lack of appetite.

MANGANESE

The greatest concentrations of this mineral are found in the pancreas, liver, pituitary, and kidneys. It is an important catalyst and a co-factor or component of many enzymes in the body. Few elements have as many metabolic functions, although the mechanisms are obscure.

Functions of Manganese.
1. Proper utilization of glucose.
2. Lipid synthesis and metabolism.
3. Cholesterol synthesis.
4. Normal pancreas function and development.
5. Prevention of sterility.

Deficiency Symptoms:
1. Weakness of ligaments and tendons.
2. Ataxia — muscular incoordination.
3. Possibly diabetes.
4. Possibly myasthenia gravis and multiple sclerosis.

IODINE

Iodine is a trace mineral limited by law to a very small dosage because of the danger of interference in normal synthesis of thyroid hormones if a large dosage of the medicinal form is administered. It is interesting to note that there is no record of any toxicity from iodine naturally occurring in a food, regardless of the amount ingested. Another facet of iodine is that it was the first nutrient designated as being essential for man.

Functions of Iodine:
1. A part of the thyroid hormones thyroxine and triiodothyronine (as such, helps to regulate many metabolic functions in the body).

Deficiency Symptoms:
1. Goiter.
2. Slow mental reactions.
3. Dry hair, brittle nails.
4. Obesity.

FLUORINE

There is much controversy regarding Fluorine, although it is an essential mineral. Most of the disagreement erupts when the chemical waste product, sodium fluoride, is proposed to be added to the drinking water as a supposed dental caries preventive.

Functions of Fluorine:
1. Increase deposition of calcium — stronger bones, etc.

Deficiency Symptoms:
1. Poor tooth development.

Symptoms of Excess:
1. Mottled teeth.
2. Inhibition of enzyme phosphatase, which assists calcium utilization.

COPPER

The need for copper in human nutrition is not often considered because so little is needed. It is however, an essential trace element and is found in all body tissues.

Function of Copper:
1. Facilitates iron absorption.
2. Involved in protein metabolism and the healing process.
3. Assists body to oxidize Vitamin C.
4. Necessary for production of RNA.
5. Essential in formation of myelin sheath.

Deficiency Symptoms:
1. General weakness — anemia.
2. Impaired respiration.
3. Skin sores.

COBALT

Cobalt is considered an essential mineral and is an integral part of vitamin B-12 (Cobalamin). Vitamin B-12 and Cobalt are so closely connected that the two terms can be used interchangeably in general reference. Animal products are our major source of this mineral, therefore vegetarian advocates are more susceptible to deficiency. All the functions and symptoms of deficiency which pertain to iron are applicable to Cobalt. An excess has been known to produce an enlarged thyroid gland, but this is very rare.

CHROMIUM

I predict that this will soon be one of the very important trace minerals in our supplemental armamentarium. Chromium is lost through many of the refining processes that our modern food undergoes.

Functions of Chromium:
1. Stimulates enzymes involved in glucose metabolism.
2. Increases effectiveness of insulin.
3. Stimulates synthesis of fatty acids.

Deficiency Symptoms:
1. Glucose intolerance particularly in diabetics.
2. Possible atherosclerosis.

COMMENT: Studies are now underway to determine why the addition of chromium to the diet seems to reverse atherosclerosis (the fact that it does is more or less scientifically established). It is my opinion that the mechanism involves the metabolism of glucose, which if improperly metabolized is converted to fats which are a major portion of the atherosclerotic plaque. If the sugar is properly metabolized, as it is in the presence of chromium, the body then has a chance to deplete the blood fat with the phospholipids and other metabolic means without a constant replenishment being furnished.

ZINC

Zinc is the second largest quantity trace mineral in the body (iron is first). Much has been learned about this mineral recently and it is emerging as one of the very essential mineral elements for good health.

Functions of Zinc:

1. Necessary for absorption and activity of vitamins, particularly the B-Complex.
2. Constituent of over 25 enzymes involved in digestion and metabolism.
3. A component of insulin.
4. Essential in the synthesis of nucleic acids.
5. Helpful in healing wounds and burns.
6. Necessary for normal prostate function.

Deficiency Symptoms:

1. Increased fatigue.
2. Susceptibility to infection, slow wound healing.
3. Prostatitis, sterility.
4. Loss of taste and smell sensitivity.
5. Possibly diabetes.

SELENIUM

Another comparative newcomer to the trace mineral arena, selenium has been accepted as an essential nutrient. Its major function is that of an antioxidant, and appears to be as much as 100 times as potent as vitamin E in this regard. Also a deficiency of this mineral would increase the body's need for vitamin E manyfold. It is found in meats and seafood primarily, although brewers yeast and certain other strains of yeast (except torula which is totally devoid of selenium) contain a goodly amount.

SULFUR

Since this mineral is so closely bound to the protein

intake, being highly concentrated therein, it is not considered possible that a deficiency could occur. Sulfur is involved in collagen formation, in the maintenance of healthy hair, fingernails, and skin and is also found in insulin.

VANADIUM

Scientiests seem to be sure that Vanadium has something to do with preventing cardiovascular disease, but as yet no precise information has been forthcoming. It is essential for normal growth and is found most abundantly in sea foods with herring and sardines having the greatest concentrations.

MOLYBDENUM

A component of several essential enzymes, Molybdenum is considered to be in such plentiful supply in cereals, dark green vegetables, and water that a deficiency would be very rare. It does assist in mobilizing iron from the reserves stored in the liver and appears to have a caries inhibiting effect.

NICKEL

Nickel activates several enzyme systems and is highly concentrated in ribonucleic acid, but the real role it plays in human nutrition is not clear at this time. Its primary source in the diet is vegetables.

TIN

We are aware that tin is necessary as a growth factor, but

the mechanism is not known. Trace amounts are widely found in both the plant and animal kingdom so deficiencies are not known.

SILICON

The most recent addition to the list of trace minerals known to be essential, silicon is needed for normal growth and bone development. It is the most abundant mineral on this earth, therefore a deficiency is unlikely.

ALUMINUM

Aluminum is a trace mineral element, but it can be injurious. Foods cooked in aluminum utensils may absorb minute quantities of the mineral. There is no known use for this mineral in the body.

Toxic Symptoms:
1. Constipation, colic, nausea, loss of appetite.
2. Twitching of leg muscles.
3. Excessive perspiration — loss of energy.
4. Motor nerve paralysis and localized numbness.

CADMIUM

Another toxic trace mineral element which will take the place of the essential mineral Zinc in the storage systems of the body. Thus, a diet deficiency in Zinc will allow the Cadmium levels to rise and a toxic state can ensue. Certain researchers feel that the specific result of an elevated Cadmium level is hypertension. Cadmium is most commonly found in coffee and tea — five or more cups of either will double the normal intake.

LEAD

LEAD POISONING IS PROBABLY THE MOST RAPID-LY INCREASING ENVIRONMENTAL RELATED DIS-EASE WE SEE TODAY! Smoking increases your daily lead intake by 25 percent — so don't blame it all on the smog. Lead replaces deficient calcium in the bone, so a high calcium diet will help prevent such a deposition. Algin from kelp and pectin will also help prevent the absorption of lead. Vitamin A and C help to prevent tissue from the damage that can result from overdosage of lead. So does chromium.

Toxic Symptoms:
1. Abdominal colic.
2. Hyperactivity in children.
3. Tired, run-down feeling; lack of ambition.
4. Nervousness, depression, apathy.
5. Psychoneuroses.
6. Dizziness, headaches.
7. Brain damage.
8. Neuromuscular diseases — Multiple Sclerosis.
9. Paralysis.

MERCURY

Mercury is definitely a toxic mineral to man. The most toxic form is methyl mercury which is found in many lakes and streams due to the dumping of this waste from manufacturing plants. The algae become contaminated with it and the fish that eat the algae are then even more contaminated because of their great consumption of algae. Nature has provided fish with certain protections, and if the fish has an adequate supply of selenium, the resulting mercury selinate is not toxic. Some fungicides contain mercury which, if sprayed upon the food, will eventually

337

contaminate man. Some medicines still contain mercury chloride, which is potentially toxic. Symptoms of mercury poisoning are: tremor, dementia, loss of ability to speak, paralysis, kidney failure, diarrhea.

ESSENTIAL MINERAL ELEMENTS FOR MAN

Calcium	Zinc
Phosphorus	Fluorine
Magnesium	Cobalt
Potassium	Molybdenum
Sodium	Selenium
Chlorine	Chromium
Iron	Nickel
Iodine	Tin
Copper	Vanadium
Manganese	Silicon
Sulfur	

So we end our discussion of minerals. That greatest lesson I can give you regarding these substances is their total integration and interdependence upon one another. It is wrong in my opinion, to diagnose and treat a single deficiency of either a vitamin or mineral. In the first place, the diagnosis may be correct but the nutrient may not be the classical deficiency — example: ANEMIA — IRON. We are sure of at least several nutrients which may produce anemia if they are lacking either in the diet or in the body to absorb and utilize them.

The safest and most rational approach to this situation is to support the total nutrition of the patient, both from a food standpoint and a food supplement viewpoint. All the nutrients should be included, then if a deficiency still exists, the symptoms should stand out so you can readily determine other specifics which must be added. This may be due to *biochemical individuality* and explains why the same nutritional approach can lead to success in seemingly unrelated conditions.

I have seen this happen so often, particularly in arthritis and diabetes where I have observed complete remissions of both on the identical program. It is also the main reason I do not use fragmented nutrition.

MINIMUM DAILY AMOUNTS THAT SHOULD BE PRESENT IN A GOOD FOOD SUPPLEMENT

Calcium	1000mg
Magnesium	400mg
Potassium	99mg
Phosphorus	150mg
Iron	20mg
Iodine	.225mg
Copper	2mg
Zinc	20mg
Chromium	.5mg
Manganese	20mg
Selenium	20mcg

This is not to say that a particular individual may not have a greater need for one particular mineral, but as I indicated in the chapter on Vitamins, if you take a good supplement which combines the above with the suggested potencies of vitamins as outlined in that chapter, the deficiencies — if any remain — should pop out like a sore thumb. Remember that both work together at all times to create abundant health.

NOTE: It is possible that under certain intimidations by the FDA, manufacturers may not include one or more of the above minerals. This does not in any way negate the need of the body for them, nor should it be considered an indication that they are toxic — particularly at the levels suggested above. Remember that any substance can be toxic at certain levels, regardless of how essential it may be. The above are considered rational and safe in my opinion.

CARBOHYDRATE
INTOLERANT
DIET PROGRAM

Early Mini-Meal .... Choice of allowable fruit.
(Upon Rising)

Breakfast .... Six ounces tomato juice, one or two eggs with choice of meat, cheese or cottage cheese. ONLY ONE slice of whole grain bread (not essential). No cold cereals allowed.

Mid-Morning Mini-Meal .... Eight ounces multiple source protein drink.**

Lunch .... Meat, fish, eggs, or cheese; vegetables as desired, permissible salads, beverage.

Mid-Afternoon Mini-Meal .. Eight ounces multiple source protein drink OR fresh fruit or vegetable juice.

**Pre-Dinner Appetite
Stabilizer** .... Six ounces vegetable juice.

Dinner .... Soup if desired (not thickened with flour), vegetables, portion of meat, fish, or poultry; one slice of whole grain bread with plenty of butter if desired, beverage.

Bedtime Mini-Meal .... Six to eight ounces of multiple source protein drink.

NOTE: At least 2/3 of the daily intake should be consumed before mid-afternoon. It is not wise to eat a large dinner.

NOTE: Some form of daily exercise is highly recommended — bicycle riding, badminton, tennis, jogging, isometrics, weight lifting, square dancing, calisthenics, etc.

THIS DIET WILL BE AS SUCCESSFUL AS YOU ARE FAITHFUL IN FOLLOWING IT.

**Your doctor will recommend the protein concentrate for you that will be used for your protein drink. Tomato or V-8 juice is an excellent base liquid for this health builder.

SELECTION CHART

CHOICE GROUP
MEAT .... Veal, beef, lamb, fish, poultry are the best choices. Ham, bacon, sausage and other processed meats should be eliminated.

FRUITS .... Apricots, apples, berries, melons, peaches, pears, pineapple, tangerines, grapefruit, oranges, cantaloupe, strawberries, watermelon, plums.

JUICES .... Any unsweetened fruit or vegetable juice, except grape or prune juice. Best fresh.

VEGETABLES .... Any vegetable except those listed below.

BEVERAGES .... Herb tea, cereal coffee substitute. No sugar added.

DESSERTS .... Fruits — preferrably eaten 3 hours after meal.

NOTE: Fruits should be raw or cooked without sugar. If you use canned, be sure they are packed in water. Best raw.

AVOID GROUP

ALCOHOLIC AND SOFT DRINKS	Wines, cordials, cocktails, beer, whiskey, cola drinks, pop of all kinds, gingerale, club soda.
VEGETABLES	Hominy, rice, yams, potato (except raw or baked twice weekly), corn, dried beans.
JUICES	Grape juice and prune juice.
PREPARED FOODS	White flour bakery products, spaghetti, macaroni, noodles, gravies.
BEVERAGES	Coffee and tea.
DESSERTS	Candy and other sugar sweets, such as cake, pie, pastries, custard, jello, ice cream, sherbets, puddings.

CLASSIFICATION OF FOODS
(According to Carbohydrate Content)

VEGETABLES

3 PERCENT	6 PERCENT	15 PERCENT	20 PERCENT	25 PERCENT
Asparagus	Beans, string	Artichokes	Beans, dried	Rice, boiled
Bean sprouts	Beets	Beans, Kidney	Beans, Lima	Potato, sweet
Beet greens	Brussel sprouts	Hominy	Corn	Yams
Broccoli	Carrots	Oyster plant	Potato, white	
Cabbage	Chives	Parsnips		
Cauliflower	Collards	Peas, green		
Celery	Dandelion			
Chard, Swiss	greens			
Cucumber	Eggplant			
Endive	Kale			
Lettuce	Kohlrabi			
Mushrooms	Leeks			
Mustard	Okra			
greens	Onions			
Radishes	Parsley			
Sauerkraut	Peppers, red			
Spinach	Pimento			
Squash	Pumpkin			
Tomatoes	Rutabagas			
Tomato juice	Turnips			
Turnip greens				
Water cress				

FRUITS

3 PERCENT	6 PERCENT	15 PERCENT	20 PERCENT	25 PERCENT
Cantaloupe	Apricots	Apples	Bananas	
Rhubarb	Blackberries	Blueberries	Figs	
Strawberries	Cranberries	Cherries	Prunes	
Watermelon	Currants	Grapes		
	Gooseberries	Kumquats		
	Grapefruit	Loganberries		
	Guava	Mangoes		
	Melons	Mulberries		
	Lemons	Pears		
	Limes	Pineapple		
	Oranges	Pomegranates		
	Papayas			
	Peaches			
	Plums			
	Raspberries			
	Tangerines			

In making your choice of vegetables, you may use all the 3% and 6% selections you wish every day. Twice weekly, choose one from the 15%, 20%, or 25% group as a change.

In making your choice of fruits, it is desirable that you limit the amount to one 3% selection during the first days of your diet. As you progress, other choices can be made.

Creative Restoration Diet

THIS MESSAGE IS FOR YOU!

It is a health program designed for modern living with a great deal of study and practical clinical experience, resulting in this concise and precision-engineered schedule. Any program can only be as effective as its application. Anything worth doing is worth doing well, so why not make it a real challenge to put it to work for a mere 30 days of your life — and in return have a chance at increased health, the greatest wealth of all?

INCOMPATIBLE WITH THIS PROGRAM

Certain habits are incompatible with your search for health. You cannot build with one hand while tearing down with the other and expect to fashion a monument. The following are incompatible with good health:

1. *Consumption of alcohol.* This has been scientifically proven to destroy brain as well as liver cells.
2. *Smoking.* So much evidence has been presented we need not elaborate, but specifically it is carcinogenic and destroys vitamin C.
3. *Over-consumption of coffee and tea.* Both of these contain habit-forming drugs and are deleterious to the central nervous system. You may substitute herb teas or cereal beverages (health food stores).

345

UNDERSTANDING THE
CREATIVE RESTORATION DIET

This is a recommended method of eating foods to induce you to 'automatically' improve your diet. *It Must Be Understood,* not just blindly followed. You must learn to lead your own way. Unlike the dull, restricted menu-type diet which requires discipline to enforce, this educational approach can be interesting. It encourages a greater, rather than lesser variety of foods, thus both taste and appetite are more likely to be satisfied. There is also a great satisfaction in being able to select foods by reason of good judgment and common sense, rather than by the usual hit or miss method.

Therefore, please read the following information carefully. If you understand why you are asked to follow certain Rules and Guidelines, it will be much easier to gain your cooperation. It merely takes plain common sense and a wisp of willpower. Your conscience should become your guide. Since this diet consists primarily of vegetables, meat, cheese, fish, poultry, and fruit, it is high in minerals, especially Potassium, an essential mineral of prime importance in the body chemistry. Because it is high in fiber foods, which are both cleansing and speed up the tract time, it encourages a favorable intestinal environment. It is intended to eliminate a high proportion of so-called "empty calorie" foods, so it should have an excellent *weight normalization* influence.

Naturally, all of the foods which one should not eat cannot be mentioned. Only the major classifications are mentioned in this regard, listing a few categories only. The guidelines for food combinations are few and easy to follow. Emphasis is placed upon the positive "what to eat" nature of dieting. It is a diet you can believe in because it is deemed to be right, founded in truth, rather than fancy or statistics.

Basic rules to follow are listed at end of this chapter. These should be learned and practiced until they become matters of habit.

GENERAL PRINCIPLES

Regarding White Flour and White Sugar Products —

Not only are white flour and sugar products devoid of their natural occurring vitamins and minerals, but the less desirable calories are concentrated until they become little more than pure starch and carbohydrate. Why is this abuse of Nature's stores brought about?

In the case of white flour, shelf-life is the main reason. All commercial white flour is processed so that it can be stored for long periods of time. To make this possible, most of the 'life' is removed from the whole wheat berries. Since the oil is removed, it cannot turn rancid. Everything subject to oxidation has been removed. If it were not so, spoilage would be very rapid, often within a period of a few days.

White sugar is refined for another reason. In its liquid form as cane juice, it would ferment rapidly and would require refrigeration from cane field to user. Obviously, this would not serve commercial purposes. Granulated sugar did! But the attendant loss of vitamins and minerals, plus the intensive concentration of purified carbohydrate, made a mixture too rich to handle by your body, much like the carburetor on your car when too much gas is mixed with the air.

An important feature of the Creative Restoration Diet is to *eat maximum quantities of live foods and eliminate purified foods.* White flour products and white sugar products are dead foods (no enzymes and most or all of the vitamins and minerals removed) and are purified substances which the body finds difficult to adapt to normal metabolism.

It is comparatively simple to eliminate much white sugar from the diet simply by not eating candy, pastries and so forth made of white sugar. However, many find it difficult to eliminate all white flour products such as bread, bakery rolls, paste foods (macaroni, spaghetti, pizza and the like). The elimination of white flour products is essential, however, if the fullest benefits are to be obtained from the Creative Restoration Diet.

Regarding the Use of Uncooked Foods —

Let's look at your diet from the aspect of how much of it consists of uncooked or raw foods. Many people go days on end with no more raw food than a smattering of lettuce or an occasional glass of fruit juice. The remainder of their diet is completely cooked! *The eating of fresh, raw foods daily should never be left to chance.* Two outstanding all-season foods are recommended as always being available:
1. Tomatoes and Tomato Juice
2. Raw Cabbage

Although raw tomatoes are usually best, canned tomatoes, without presevatives added, are on the list of acceptable foods. Tomatoes are one of the few vegetables which lend themselves well to the canning process. In fact, because tomatoes are canned at the height of their natural perfection, the food value can be higher than the hot house varieties sold in off-seasons. The same applies to tomato juice, with both offering rich sources of Potassium, and Vitamins A, B, and C.

Salads made with raw cabbage instead of lettuce can be one of the greatest taste surprises you have ever had. Cabbage in raw form is one of our richest sources of essential vitamins and minerals. It stores as well, if not better, than any other raw food, keeping its nutrients beneath its protective wrapper in the leaves. *It is indispensable to the success of this diet that a high quality raw food be included in the diet daily.* Tomato and cabbage have been sugested — if at all possible, I use one cupful of raw cabbage with a little raw potato or jicama or water chestnut mixed in every day — raw carrots, cauliflower, sprouts, celery, etc. are almost always available and can be used to excellent advantage.

Regarding Use of Meat Products —

Meats, such as veal, beef, lamb, and chicken are good sources of protein. However, even though the protein intake is adequate insofar as quantity is concerned, quality is an even more important point to consider. Incomplete proteins leave out pieces of the 'building block' mechanism, and like a jigsaw puzzle with pieces missing, the whole picture suffers. This can be a good reason to supplement the diet with a multiple-source protein product to assure an adequate amino acid supply and balance.

Also in regard to protein ingestion, its breakdown into amino acids is essential to its utilization. This is called the process of digestion. If digestion fails to liquify the meat (protein), spoilage can occur in the intestinal tract — a process called putrefication. Effects of putrefaction in the gastrointestinal tract are bad breath, foul odored stool and a general decrease in energy. This is a good reason to supplement the diet with an appropriate digestive enzyme product, both facilitating breakdown of the protein and preventing putrefaction.

Contrary to some opinions, the grinding of meat into small particles, e.g., hamburger, does not increase its digestibility. On the other hand, grinding of meat can have deleterious effects. Ground meat spoils rapidly at room temperature, whole meat does not; in fact, aging of whole meat can make it more tender by a sort of 'predigestion' which occurs.

It is postulated that nucleic acids are released when meat is ground, coming out with the meat juices, apparently making spoilage very fast by this means. Similar action may occur when ground meat is introduced into the intestinal tract. There the temperature is ideal for rapid spoilage. *This is particularly applicable if there is insufficient hydrochloric acid in the stomach,* as HCl acts as an intestinal antiseptic to inhibit fermentation and putrefaction which might otherwise occur. Here, again, a proper digestive aid containing hydrochloric acid sources may be used to a distinct advantage.

Note: Preserved meats, such as weiners and sausages, do not have as much tendency to putrefaction, since they contain anti-putrefactive chemicals (usually nitrites and/or nitrates) which work both inside and ouside the body to produce this effect. However, for the same reason they are not desirable from a nutritional viewpoint. It has been determined that these substances inhibit enzymes in the body, produce liver and kidney disease, as well as being possibly carcinogenic.

Regarding the Use of Sugar and Protein and/or Fat Combinations

One of the little known deleterious effects of refined sugar is its reaction in the gastrointestinal tract with protein and/or fat combinations. First of all, let us establish that concentrated carbohydrates (sugars) stay in the stomach for only a short period of time since very little digestion is necessary. On the other hand, protein remains in the stomach for extended periods of time (up to 5 hours) because much activity must take place before the proteins can be passed on to the small intestine for absorption. Some fats also are broken down in the stomach and the presence of fat in the stomach slows down the production of hydrochloric acid which further delays the time of departure of stomach contents. When concentrated carbohydrates are mixed with protein or protein/fat combinations, the sugars tend to ferment in the stomach, producing gas. Adequate hydrochloric acid will prevent this to some extent, but the major cause of stomach gas is improper combining of food groups. Too many Americans are accustomed to finishing off a good protein meal with sweet desserts. For best nutrition, concentrated sweets should be eaten on an empty stomach — this includes fruits, fruit juices, etc.

There are many sugar protein combinations which may be easily avoided if one is on the alert; an outstanding example is eggs with orange juice. The fact that many foods contain a combination of protein and carbohydrate must be taken into consideration — such natural combinations rarely give much trouble as it is concentration of carbohydrate which produces the deleterious effects, these being proportional to the quantity present.

Regarding the Use of Fiber Foods in the Diet —

As a natural laxative, without griping, diarrhea, or any of the other complaints we have about most other laxatives, dietary fiber has no equal. Although many are not aware, they suffer from extremely slow movement of the digestive tract. There are many consequences of such slow tract time: 1. Intestinal gas because of the fermentation of starches and sugars. 2. Diverticulosis due to the large amounts of fecal material pushing against the wall of the intestine producing little sacs or pouches which then fill with waste material. This is ideal circumstance for more putrefaction to occur which then discharges noxious matter into the tract which may be absorbed into the blood stream. 3. Hemorrhoids and Varicosities can be blamed, at least in part to the pressure exerted by the large amounts of material collected in the intestinal tract on the pelvic veins creating back pressure which balloons the veins in the hemorrhoidal plexus and in the leg.

It would be a very apathetic individual indeed, who would not see the advantages of consuming some form of dietary fiber each and every day in order to help prevent the above from becoming a reality in his or her life. The Creative Restoration Diet suggests that one-half cup of wheat bran flakes be consumed every day. These are not the processed bran flake cereals found in the supermarket but 100% bran flakes usually found in health food stores. They can be mixed with granola, yogurt, salads, casseroles, etc. Bran or dietary fiber should not be referred to as 'roughage' but rather as 'softage' because it becomes a very soft, water filled bulk in the intestines. The use of bran remedies the lack of fiber in a diet made up primarily of proteins (which contain very little fiber) and comparatively few raw fruits and vegetables.

Regarding the Use of Common Salt in the Diet —

People who use as much salt as they like may excrete nine times as much potassium, an essential mineral, as those on salt restricted diets. Actually, Americans frequently consume 20 to 25 times as much salt as estimated sodium requirements recommend. If this is not counterbalanced with increased potassium intake, a borderline potassium deficiency state is easily brought about. Salt substitutes, mostly made up of potassium chloride, are often too bitter for anyone to stick with their use. We are fortunate to have a new 60-40 mixture of sodium and potassium chlorides on the market. This satisfies flavor requirements and you need not worry about the loss of potassium from using sodium chloride alone. This formula is available in most supermarkets and health food stores.

OVERALL PICTURE
OF THE
CREATIVE RESTORATION DIET

In order to help you obtain a better idea of the recommended diet, examples of Desirable and Undesirable foods are listed. Of course, not all foods in each category can be shown, but a study of the examples given will suffice to show the type of food necessary for best results.

DESIRABLE FOODS

1. All Garden Vegetables (fresh, frozen, canned, in order of desirability)

Asparagus	Broccoli	Rutabaga	Tomato	Cabbage
Peas	Potatoes	Carrots	Yams	Celery
Parsley	Parsnips	Squash	Lettuce	Cauliflower
Chard	Corn	Sprouts	Garbanzas	String Beans

2. Meat Dishes (veal, beef, lamb, venison, elk, buffalo, fish)

Steaks	Chops	Roast	Stew	Broiled

3. Fermented Foods
Buttermilk Yogurt   Kefir   Sauerkraut   Cottage Cheese

4. Fruits, Fruit Juices, Vegetable Juices
All are acceptable — just be careful as to the combination of fruits and/or fruit juices with proteins. Fruit juices should be diluted 50%.

5. Nuts and Seeds
These are preferably in the raw state or dry roasted with little salt. They belong to the protein-fat category of foods.

6. Dietary Fiber
Wheat Bran   Rice Bran   Oatmeal   Agar-Agar   Pectin

UNDESIRABLE FOODS

1. Commercially Processed Flour Products
White Breads White Buns Biscuits White Rolls
Crackers Cookies Cakes Doughnuts
Spaghetti Macaroni Dumplings Pie Crusts

2. Commercially Processed White Sugar Products
Candy Soda Pop Pie Pudding

3. Ground or Processed Meat
Meat Loaf Hamburger Weiners Sausage Lunch Meats
Hash Chili Potted Meat
(The exception to ground meat is when you grind it fresh and immediately use it).

UNDESIRABLE FOODS (Continued)

4. Sugar — Protein Combinations

Ice Cream Chocolate Milk   Milk Shakes
Baked Beans Desserts with meals Fruits or fruit juices with
meat, eggs, cheese

BASIC RULES OF CREATIVE RESTORATION DIET

1. *Eat no foods prepared from commercially processed white flour or white sugar.*

2. *Drink at least one glass of tomato juice and eat one serving of cabbage each and every day.*

3. *Avoid the use of ground or processed meat.*

4. *Never combine high concentrations of sugar and protein at one time or at the same meal.*

5. *Include one-half cup of bran flakes in your daily diet.*

6. *Use a 60-40 mixture of sodium and potassium chlorides as salt.*

7. *Try to eat as much of your fruit and vegetables raw as circumstances permit.*

Note: The foregoing dietary recommendations are for general nutritional purposes only, and are not to be considered substitutes for any specific nutritional counsel or advice of your doctor concerning specific situations. Certain persons considered experts may disagree with one or more of the preceeding statements or recommendations.

355

The National Addiction

COFFEE

THE NOT SO WONDERFUL WORLD OF THE AROMATIC BREW — COFFEE

Both socially and privately, coffee drinking is indisputably the drink and choice among Americans. Eight out of ten adults drink it each and every day. We sip three times more of it than we do soft drinks, four times more than beer. We drink 50 times more of it than hard liquor. We take it black or creamed, sweetened or bitter, hot or iced. So much of it washes down the national gullet that the electric coffee-maker is expected to displace the trusty iron as the hottest-selling small appliance.

The beverage's place in American social life is without peer. No other drink — not even coca-cola — approaches coffee as a universal beverage in the American way of life. Coffee houses, coffee cake, coffee break are all words which have been coined to accommodate the universal addiction to this brew. It has been used to substitute for other addictions — Alcoholics Anonymous members have an average intake of 20 cups per day — although you don't have to be an ex-alcoholic to consume that much daily — many who are opposed to alcohol on religious principles see no wrong in the drinking of this beverage which can be just as addicting and health destroying as alcohol.

ADDICTION

Evidence of such addictive properties are not difficult to come by, just ask any coffee drinker what happens when he abstains for a day — the answer will usually be headaches, fatigue, stomach pains, etc. The major addictive factor in coffee is caffeine, a white crystalline alkaloid that stimulates the brain and artificially lessens fatigue. Caffeine is a poison. A sizable concentration injected into an animal's skin will kill within minutes. Injected into human muscles, it will cause paralysis. Ten grams of caffeine (the amount in 100 cups of coffee) accumulated suddenly in the human body would be lethal — resulting in death.

Fortunately, coffee ingested in the common manner is not fatal, since the kidneys work overtime to eliminate this toxin from the body and prevent its accumulation. But even these smaller caffeine doses make things happen which might cause some to reconsider.

1. After one or more cups of coffee, the stomach temperature rises 10 to 15 degrees.
2. The secretion of hydrochloric acid increases 400 percent.
3. The salivary glands double their output.
4. The heart beats faster.
5. The lungs work harder.
6. The blood vessels narrow in the brain and widen in and around the heart.
7. Metabolic rate increases.
8. Kidneys manufacture and discharge up to 100 percent more urine.

DIS-EASE CORRELATION

Psychiatrist Julius Rice declares — "Three or four cups

of coffee taken in quick succession contain sufficient caffeine to produce irritability, nervousness, tremor, headache, and heart palpitations. Double or treble this amount may cause hallucinations and possibly convulsions." There is also evidence associating coffee with bladder cancer, in fact the rate of bladder cancer among coffee drinkers is 2½ times greater than among non-coffee drinkers.

The very real risk of cancer can be documented by the fact that caffeine has been shown to cause mutations in cells in tissue cultures. A cancer cell is a mutated cell.

In 1972 and again in 1973, studies were done which implicated the consumption of coffee to myocardial infarction, a condition in which the heart muscle tissue degenerates because of a restricted blood flow. According to the study, this disease is 200% as prevalent in coffee drinkers as in non-coffee drinkers. Coffee is also the major dietary source of cadmium, a toxic mineral which has been linked with heart disease and high blood pressure.

HYPOGLYCEMIA

Another disturbing relationship to ill health is the effect coffee has on the hypoglycemic or low blood sugar victim. This disease is characterized by periods of below normal levels of blood sugar which often produce symptoms of nervousness, insomnia, lack of concentration, headaches, chest pains, fatigue, sinusitis, cold sweats, depression, shortness of breath, irritability, forgetfulness, and many others. The victim soon finds that a cup of coffee can, at least temporarily, relieve these symptoms and at their onset, heads for the pot of coffee. The mechanism of action is really quite simple; caffeine is such an irritant that it stimulates the releases of adrenal hormones to help the body defend itself against it. Among other things, these hormones are the synergist which converts glycogen (inert storage sugar) into glucose which is the form of sugar in the blood stream. Since the brain depends exclusively upon glucose for its fuel, and in the hypoglycemic state the brain is without adequate fuel, the symptoms listed above are quite logical. Just as logical is the inevitable result of such an artificial raising of the blood sugar by defensive reflex of the body — namely that of an eventual addiction to the substance with offers temporary relief — in this case coffee.

WHIPPING A TIRED HORSE

I would like to elaborate a little on the whole business of the stimulating effect of coffee. We have indicated that blood sugar can be raised by coffee, that heart rates can be increased, that gastric secretions of hydrochloric acid are quadrupled, that the lungs are stimulated, the kidneys work overtime, and changes take place in the blood vessels in the entire body. Can there be any benefit from such stimulation? I think not. After all, if we feel fatigued, the body is usually trying to tell us something — that we need rest or that we can use some food to replenish the fuel supply needed for energy. When we use a chemical substitute for either of these we are whipping a tired horse. The result will be a temporary speeding up, but eventually the horse will collapse. Sooner or later we all have to accept the laws of nature.

CAFFEINE AND YOUR BRAIN AND NERVES

Intensive tests on guinea pigs, who were given doses of caffeine, indicated that the effect of caffeine on the brain and nervous tissues of the test animals was more serious and more destructive than doses of morphine. Consider that for a moment — would you think of using small amounts of morphine every day. Obviously not, but yet another drug is a component of our national beverage. Is it possible that your nervous system could work much better without a constant bombardment with a destructive drug?

YOU DESERVE BETTER THINGS

Would you agree that everything you put into your body should be for the benefit and use of the body? Coffee does not come in such a category. It has no positive, helpful function. It furnishes no vitamins, minerals, enzymes or protein to the diet. Caffeine does create many problems which causes the body to expend much energy to over-come. It may be of interest to you to know that the average cup of tea has at least one-half the content of caffeine as coffee, cola drinks contain about 25% as much caffeine as coffee, and all chocolate contains caffeine.

There are many herb teas and coffee substitutes which can be consumed to the benefit of the body, rather than its detriment. The elimination of coffee and other caffeine con-taining substances from your diet can be one of the most important health moves you ever made.

Hidden Sugars
in Foods

"HIDDEN SUGARS" IN FOODS

Food Item	Size of Portion	Approx. sugar content in teaspoonfuls of granulated sugar
BEVERAGES		
Cola Drinks	1 (6 oz. bottle or glass)	3½
Cordials	1 (3¾ oz. glass)	1½
Ginger Ale	6 oz.	5
Hi-Ball	1 (6 oz. glass)	2½
Orange-Ade	1 (8 oz. glass)	5
Root Beer	1 (10 oz. bottle)	4½
Seven-Up	1 (6 oz. bottle or glass)	3¾
Soda Pop	1 (8 oz. bottle)	5
Sweet Cider	1 cup	6
Whiskey Sour	1 (3 oz. glass)	1½
CAKES & COOKIES		
Angel Food	1 (4 oz. piece)	7
Apple Sauce Cake	1 (4 oz. piece)	5½
Banana Cake	1 (2 oz. piece)	2
Cheese Cake	1 (4 oz. piece)	2
Chocolate Cake, Plain	1 (4 oz. piece)	6
Chocolate Cake, Iced	1 (4 oz. piece)	10
Coffee Cake	1 (4 oz. piece)	4½
Cup Cake, Iced	1	6
Fruit Cake	1 (4 oz. piece)	5
Jelly-Roll	1 (2 oz. piece)	2½
Orange Cake	1 (4 oz. piece)	4
Pound Cake	1 (4 oz. piece)	5
Sponge Cake	1 (4 oz. piece)	2
Strawberry Shortcake	1 serving	4
Brownies, unfrosted	1 (¾ oz.)	3
Chocolate Cookies	1	1½
Fig Newtons	1	5
Ginger Snaps	1	3

"HIDDEN SUGARS" IN FOODS

Food Item	Size of Portion	Approx. sugar content in teaspoonfuls of granulated sugar
Macaroons	1	6
Nut Cookies	1	1½
Oatmeal Cookies	1	2
Sugar Cookies	1	1½
Chocolate Eclair	1	7
Cream Puff	1	2
Donut, Plain	1	3
Donut, Glazed	1	6
Snail	1 (4 oz. piece)	4½

CANDIES

Food Item	Size of Portion	Approx. sugar content
Average Chocolate Milk Bar (example: Hershey bar)	1 (1½ oz.)	2½
Chewing Gum	1 stick	½
Chocolate Cream	1 piece	2
Butterscotch Chew	1 piece	1
Chocolate Mints	1 piece	2
Fudge	1 oz. square	4½
Gum Drop	1	2
Hard Candy	4 oz.	20
Lifesavers	1	1/3
Peanut Brittle	1 oz.	3½

CANNED FRUITS & JUICES

Food Item	Size of Portion	Approx. sugar content
Canned Apricots	4 halves & 1 Tbsp. syrup	3½
Canned Fruit Juice (swtnd)	½ Cup	2
Canned Peaches	2 halves & 1 Tbsp. syrup	3½
Fruit Salad	½ Cup	3½
Fruit Syrup	2 Tbsp.	2½
Stewed Fruits	½ Cup	2

DAIRY PRODUCTS

Food Item	Size of Portion	Approx. sugar content
Ice Cream	1/3 pt. (3½ oz.)	3½
Ice Cream Bar	1	1-7 depending on size
Ice Cream Cone	1	3½
Ice Cream Soda	1	5
Ice Cream Sundae	1	7
Malted Milk Shake	1 (10 oz. glass)	5

362

Food Item	Size of Portion	Approx. sugar content in teaspoonfuls of granulated sugar

JAMS & JELLIES

Food Item	Size of Portion	
Apple Butter	1 Tbsp.	1
Jelly	1 Tbsp.	4-6
Orange Marmelade	1 Tbsp.	4-6
Peach Butter	1 Tbsp.	1
Strawberry Jam	1 Tbsp.	4

DESSERTS, MISCELLANEOUS

Food Item	Size of Portion	
Apple Cobbler	½ Cup	3
Blueberry Cobbler	½ Cup	3
Custard	½ Cup	2
French Pastry	1 (4 oz. piece)	5
Jello	½ Cup	4½

"SUCROSE" CONTENT OF 24 LEADING CEREALS

Kelloggs Apple Jacks	% 52.04
Post Fruity Pebbles	48.51
Ralston Purina Cookie Crisp	45.45
Quaker King Vitamin	42.40
Post Super Sugar Crisp	42.16
Quaker Cap'n Crunch	39.09
Kellogs Frosted Flakes	39.07
General Mills Trix	37.27
General Mills Golden Grahams	29.90
Kellogs Cracklin Bran	27.50
Kelloggs Country Morning	21.85
Nabisco 100% Bran	19.77
Kelloggs Frosted Mini Wheats	19.77
C. W. Post	18.20
Quaker 100% Natural	17.09

Kretschmer Sun Country Granola
with almonds   16.82
Ralston Purina Bran Chex   14.25
Post Raisin Bran   12.97
Kelloggs 40% Bran Flakes   12.88
Kelloggs Raisin Bran   12.20
Kelloggs Rice Krispies   8.62
Wheaties   8.60
Kelloggs Corn Flakes   5.03
Cheerios   3.07

Sucrose is refined white table sugar (except when found in nature, in less than 5% of total weight) of the empty calorie type, with the vitamins and minerals refined out.

Do You Know What Happens When You Smoke?

RECENT RESEARCH HAS GIVEN US A DEEPER UNDERSTANDING OF HOW RUGGED CIGARETTE COUNTRY REALLY IS

According to John A. Yacinda, who runs a smoking withdrawal clinic for the Ventura County Health Department in California, the question teen-agers most often ask about smoking is "How long does it take for cigarettes to harm you?" His answer: "About three seconds."

Or less. The fact is that the instant you inhale cigarette smoke, that rich country flavor goes to work — on your heart, your lungs, your whole body. It starts your heart pounding an extra 15 to 25 beats per minute, raises your blood pressure by 10 to 20 points. It corrodes the delicate membranes of your lips and palate. In your lungs, it chokes the airways and rots the air sacs, leaving a residue of cancer-causing chemicals. It deposits these and other dangerous poisons in your stomach, kidneys, bladder. All of this happens with *every* cigarette you smoke; no smoker is immune.

And when you exhale, up to 90 percent of that true tobacco taste stays with you — in the form of billions of microscopic particles comprising 1200 chemicals. In this balanced blend of fine aromas are acids, glycerol, glycol, alcohols, aldehydes, ketones, aliphatic and aromatic hydrocarbons, phenols. None is a health food; many will do you harm.

365

Insidious CO. For years some scientists scoffed that it wasn't possible for one substance — smoke — to attack so many parts of the body in so many ways. Research has proved, however, that tobacco smoke isn't a single substance. At least 50 percent of the country-fresh flavor you inhale is gas — 20 different noxious vapors, including acrolein, hydrocyanic acid, nitric oxide, nitrogen dioxide, acetone and ammonia. And now science is zeroing in on one that's even deadlier: colorless, odorless, *lethal carbon monoxide (CO).*

Present in cigarette smoke in a concentration 640 times the safe level in industrial plants, this insidious poison has 200 times the affinity for your red blood cells that life-giving oxygen does — and those cells are designed to carry oxygen throughout your body. Therefore, in a smoker, blood is transporting five to ten times more life-denying CO than is normal. His body is forced to compensate by making more red cells.

Mainly, CO prevents red cells from picking up enough oxygen; but it also inhibits them from giving up oxygen as fast as your tissues demand. Because of this whipsaw CO effect, cigarette country is always about 8000 feet above sea level. A cigarette smoker who lives at zero altitude is getting as little oxygen as someone who's nearly two miles high.

There's no age limit on the effect, either. A teen-age novice smoker may feel winded under mild stress, even if he smokes only five or six cigarettes per day. Every smoker who is a sportsman will find himself out of breath more quickly than his non-smoking competitors. And this is only one of the less deadly results of CO. Consider what happens when its effects join up with those of nicotine, a poison found in nature exclusively in tobacco.

New studies indicate that a pregnant woman who smokes is smoking for two: nicotine constricts blood vessels in her unborn child, cutting down on fetal blood flow, while CO cuts down the amount of oxygen in the reduced blood supply. The fetus just can't get enough blood or oxygen to grow as fast as it normally would. The babies of mothers who smoke during pregnancy weigh an average of six ounces less at birth than those of non-smoking mothers. Smoking mothers also have more miscarriages and still-births, and more of their babies die within one month of birth.

Hapless Hearts. It's the nicotine in cigarettes that gives you a "lift" — it lifts your blood pressure, your heartbeat and the amount of blood pumped by your heart. It does this by releasing substances known as catecholamines (the main one is adrenalin) into your tissues. The catecholamines push your heart so hard that it requires more blood in its coronary arteries to keep up with the demand. Healthy hearts rise to the occasion. But in people with coronary-artery disease, the hard-working heart does not get enough additional blood.

The adrenalin released by nicotine also hits fat cells all over your body, causing them to pour free fatty acids into your blood. Every time you smoke, the level of free fatty acids in your blood goes up. These elevated levels of fatty acids may have an accelerating effect on clotting. Some studies have shown that platelets, a clotting factor in the blood, also becomes more adhesive in smokers.

Moreover, animal studies show that carbon monoxide makes artery walls more permeable to fatty substances. This may be one of the mechanisms leading to the deposit of fatty plaques which narrow arterial passages — athero-sclerosis.

Smoking doesn't cause all the heart attacks in the United States. But one scientist calculates that cigarettes alone are responsible for about 188,000 of the one million U.S. deaths from heart and artery disease each year.

Tar Struck. What produces most of the flavor in your cigarettes is those billions of chemical particles mentioned earlier. Condensed from smoke, they form viscous, smelly tar. A pack-a-day smoker each year inhales about a full cup — eight ounces — of tar in his smoke that satisfies.

Even as it pours tar into your lungs, smoke neutralizes the lungs' defenses: mucus, to trap dirt and microbes; cilia, tiny hairlike structures lining the airways, beating steadily to move the mucus toward the throat; and macrophages, hard-working vacuum-cleaner cells which gather and dispose of harmful substances. The cigarette smoke you gulp directly into your lungs produces excess mucus while slowing down and eventually stopping the cilia, and hampering the macrophages' ability to digest foreign matter.

In that tar — against which you now can't defend yourself — animal studies show that there are about 30 chemicals which help cause cancer. Several are "complete carcinogens," which means that they can start malignant tumors all by themselves. One such is beta-naphthylamine, a specific cause of bladder cancer in human beings and so powerful that many countries have restricted its manufacture (it's used in dyes). A medical researcher has calculated that 35 percent of bladder cancers in the United States are caused by cigarettes, resulting in 3,100 deaths a year.

But tar itself is a more powerful cancer-causing agent than the sum of its parts. Wherever it touches tissue, it produces abnormal cells. These aren't cancer, but it is among these deformed cells that cancers start. In pipe and cigar smokers who don't generally inhale, the common smoking-caused cancer areas are lip, tongue, mouth, larynx and esophagus. In cigarette smokers who inhale, the cancers also include lung, bladder and pancreas. Lung cancer is more than 90-percent fatal. Some 5,000 of the 69,000 annual U.S. deaths from lung cancer are caused by cigarettes. (Most of the dead are men, but the percentage of women is on the rise.

Ravaged Lungs. Cigarettes cause other lung diseases, which let you smoke yourself to death more slowly. Most smokers know well that first-thing-in-the-morning coughing spell. It starts the day because during the night your anesthetized cilia began to wake up and move the mucus. As smoking continues, the cough becomes chronic. Steady hacking and spitting are the symptoms of chronic bronchitis. Over-production of mucus caused by this disease provides a breeding ground for bacteria while reducing the lungs' ability to fight off infection — one reason why smokers get more colds and other respiratory infections. Chronic bronchitis can kill, too.

Chronic bronchitis and its steady companion, emphysema of which the U.S. Surgeon General says, cigarettes are the most important cause — kill about 30,000 Americans a year. There is good reason to believe that 99 percent of heavy cigarette smokers (more than a pack a day) have some emphysema, a disease that destroys the lungs' air sacs. Recently a pathologist studied the lungs of some 1800 deceased men and women and classified them by the amount of emphysema apparent. More than 99 percent of those who had smoked heavily had the disease, and in 19 percent it was far advanced; 90 percent of the non-smokers had no emphysema, and there wasn't a single advanced case among them. Even among coal miners and others exposed to lung-damaging dust, smoking plays a significant part in death from emphysema.

"Lung cancer is a comparatively merciful death." says one doctor. "With emphysema you start gasping, and you may gasp for 15 years." It creeps up on smokers. We all start with about 100 square yards of interior lung surface. But we almost never need all of this; most of us live on a small part of our lung capacity (about 20 percent of it). The first hint a smoker gets of emphysema is when he finds himself out of breath after a small exertion. He may think this is an early warning; it isn't. It means that most of his lung reserve has been destroyed.

Even when warned, many smokers bravely refuse to give up cigarettes until it is too late. Visit the respiratory ward of you local hospital and you'll see them — never more than a few yards from their oxygen tanks and respirators, their entire lives devoted to one thing: breathing.

The Only Solution. The list of smoking-related diseases goes on yet further. Smokers have more gastric ulcers than non-smokers, and take longer to heal; more peridontal disease, which attacks teeth and gums, and more trench mouth; more severe upper respiratory infections. And evidence is beginning to show that cigarette smoke attacks the central nervous system.

The damage is "dose-related." Each cigarette does some harm. Each additional smoke repeats the insult. Eventually these incessant attacks on the body may turn into disease. With about one million puffs, or 100,000 cigarettes — a pack a day for 15 years — smokers edge into the lung-cancer danger zone.

There's no such thing as a safe level of smoking. But since the harm *is* dose-related, research shows that cutting down on the number of cigarettes, and smoking those with efficient filters and less tar and nicotine, will reduce the risk of serious illness. However, the real payoff comes from quitting.

Liver-Kidney-Bowel Cleansing Fast

LIVER-KIDNEY-BOWEL CLEANSING FAST

One of the most important factors in any disease condition is the detoxification of the body. It should also follow that such a detoxification can be an excellent means of preventing disease and promoting good health. The following is a simple three day program which accomplishes detoxification of the major organs involved in retaining toxins in the body.

Materials needed:
1. From 12 to 16 lemons daily depending on size.
2. From 2 to 6 whole beets daily, including root and top.
3. From 2 to 3 quarts distilled water daily.
4. Small container of honey.
5. Bottle of dietary fiber tablets.

FIRST DAY: One and one-half cups freshly squeezed lemon juice mixed with two quarts of distilled water and a little honey for palatibility. This will be your total intake of fluid and food for the day, so you may sip on it constantly during the day. In addition, juice sufficient from whole beets (tops and root) to make two fluid ounces of juice and consume this. Take eight dietary tablets in the morning and eight in the afternoon with full ten ounce glasses of lemon mixture.

SECOND DAY: Repeat lemon-distilled water-honey mixture and the eight dietary fiber tablets twice daily. Increase beet juice to four ounces.

THIRD DAY: Repeat lemon-distilled water-honey mixture and the eight dietary fiber tablets twice daily. Increase beet juice to six ounces.

This is the end of the concentrated detoxifying, but the first week after this program is extremely important regarding the lasting benefits. The following suggestions as to eating should be observed.

FOURTH & FIFTH DAY: Stop using the lemon-distilled water-honey mixture, but continue the dietary fiber tablets. Drink all you wish of tomato juice, carrot juice, grape juice (dilute grape juice with about one third spring water) or other vegetable or fruit juices. Eliminate citrus juices. Consume all the fresh spring water you wish.

SIXTH & SEVENTH DAY: Add raw fruits and vegetables to your regime, maintaining dietary fiber tablet intake and juices as desired.

EIGHTH DAY: Add yogurt and/or cottage cheese, continue dietary fiber.

NINTH DAY: Add lightly steamed vegetables, reduce dietary fiber to 12.

TENTH DAY: Add small portion of meat to one meal.

ELEVENTH DAY FORWARD: Follow Creative Restoration Diet; adjust dietary fiber tablets according to physician's advice.

372

NOTE: Food supplements may be continued throughout the entire program if desired, also kidney stimulants such as the herbs Buchu, Uva Ursi, Juniper, etc. can be used to promote the flow of urine. *A word of caution:* It is extremely important that the specified quantity of liquid is taken into the system each day; the success of your fast depends on strict adherence to the rules without exceptions. If by any chance nausea is produced or the beet juice should prove too distasteful, the dilution with a small amount of celery or apple juice is permitted. It is to be emphasized that this does not reduce the stated amounts of beet juice.

ALTERNATE LIVER CLEANSING PROGRAM

If you find beets totally unpalatable or fresh lemons unavailable, the following program may be used.

Buy *pure* concentrated lemon juice and make up the lemon mixture of 1½ cups equivalent lemon juice (from concentrate) and mix with 2 quarts of distilled water *each day*. Purchase a combination of the following herbs from your health food store and take 4 tablets the first day, 6 tablets the second day and 8 tablets the third day. In addition, use 8 dietary fiber tablets twice daily. After the third day continue the program as outlined.

Herb Formula: Garlic, Mandrake, Quassia, Black Cohosh, Chaparral, Foenugreek, Red Sage and Golden Seal.

—W—

—X—

—Y—

—Z—